ADEQUACY OF EVIDENCE FOR PHYSICAL ACTIVITY GUIDELINES DEVELOPMENT

WORKSHOP SUMMARY

Carol West Suitor and Vivica I. Kraak, *Rapporteurs*

Food and Nutrition Board
Board on Population Health and Public Health Practice

INSTITUTE OF MEDICINE
OF THE NATIONAL ACADEMIES

THE NATIONAL ACADEMIES PRESS
Washington, D.C.
www.nap.edu

THE NATIONAL ACADEMIES PRESS • 500 Fifth Street, N.W. • Washington, DC 20001

NOTICE: The project that is the subject of this report was approved by the Governing Board of the National Research Council, whose members are drawn from the councils of the National Academy of Sciences, the National Academy of Engineering, and the Institute of Medicine. The members of the planning committee responsible for the workshop were chosen for their special competences and with regard for appropriate balance.

The study was supported by Contract No. HHSP23320042509XI, Task Order No. 07 between the National Academy of Sciences and the United States Department of Health and Human Services. Any opinions, findings, conclusions, or recommendations expressed in this publication are those of the authors and do not necessarily reflect the views of the organizations or agencies that provided support for the project.

International Standard Book Number-13 978-0-309-10402-9
International Standard Book Number-10 0-309-10402-5

Additional copies of this report are available from the National Academies Press, 500 Fifth Street, N.W., Box 285, Washington, DC 20055. Call (800) 624-6242 or (202) 334-3313 (in the Washington metropolitan area), Internet, http://www.nap.edu.

For more information about the Institute of Medicine, visit the IOM home page at: **www.iom.edu.**

Printed in the United States of America.

Suggested citation: Institute of Medicine (IOM). 2007. *Adequacy of evidence for physical activity guidelines development: Workshop summary.* Washington, DC: The National Academies Press.

The serpent has been a symbol of long life, healing, and knowledge among almost all cultures and religions since the beginning of recorded history. The serpent adopted as a logotype by the Institute of Medicine is a relief carving from ancient Greece, now held by the Staatliche Museen in Berlin.

"Knowing is not enough; we must apply.
Willing is not enough; we must do."
—Goethe

INSTITUTE OF MEDICINE
OF THE NATIONAL ACADEMIES

Advising the Nation. Improving Health.

THE NATIONAL ACADEMIES

Advisers to the Nation on Science, Engineering, and Medicine

The **National Academy of Sciences** is a private, nonprofit, self-perpetuating society of distinguished scholars engaged in scientific and engineering research, dedicated to the furtherance of science and technology and to their use for the general welfare. Upon the authority of the charter granted to it by the Congress in 1863, the Academy has a mandate that requires it to advise the federal government on scientific and technical matters. Dr. Ralph J. Cicerone is president of the National Academy of Sciences.

The **National Academy of Engineering** was established in 1964, under the charter of the National Academy of Sciences, as a parallel organization of outstanding engineers. It is autonomous in its administration and in the selection of its members, sharing with the National Academy of Sciences the responsibility for advising the federal government. The National Academy of Engineering also sponsors engineering programs aimed at meeting national needs, encourages education and research, and recognizes the superior achievements of engineers. Dr. Wm. A. Wulf is president of the National Academy of Engineering.

The **Institute of Medicine** was established in 1970 by the National Academy of Sciences to secure the services of eminent members of appropriate professions in the examination of policy matters pertaining to the health of the public. The Institute acts under the responsibility given to the National Academy of Sciences by its congressional charter to be an adviser to the federal government and, upon its own initiative, to identify issues of medical care, research, and education. Dr. Harvey V. Fineberg is president of the Institute of Medicine.

The **National Research Council** was organized by the National Academy of Sciences in 1916 to associate the broad community of science and technology with the Academy's purposes of furthering knowledge and advising the federal government. Functioning in accordance with general policies determined by the Academy, the Council has become the principal operating agency of both the National Academy of Sciences and the National Academy of Engineering in providing services to the government, the public, and the scientific and engineering communities. The Council is administered jointly by both Academies and the Institute of Medicine. Dr. Ralph J. Cicerone and Dr. Wm. A. Wulf are chair and vice chair, respectively, of the National Research Council.

www.national-academies.org

PLANNING COMMITTEE ON THE ADEQUACY OF EVIDENCE FOR PHYSICAL ACTIVITY GUIDELINES DEVELOPMENT

WILLIAM L. HASKELL *(Chair)*, Stanford Prevention Research Center, Stanford University School of Medicine, Stanford, CA
RODNEY K. DISHMAN, Kinesiology Department, University of Georgia, Athens
JOSEPH E. DONNELLY, Energy Balance Laboratory and The Center for Physical Activity and Weight Management, The Schiefelbusch Institute for Lifespan Studies, The University of Kansas, Lawrence
BRUCE H. JONES, Epidemiology and Disease Surveillance, U.S. Army Center for Health Promotion and Preventive Medicine, Aberdeen, MD
MIRIAM E. NELSON, John Hancock Center for Physical Activity and Nutrition, The Gerald J. and Dorothy R. Friedman School of Nutrition Science and Policy, Tufts University, Boston, MA

Consultant and Rapporteur
CAROL WEST SUITOR, Northfield, VT

Staff
VIVICA I. KRAAK, Study Director
LINDA D. MEYERS, Director, Food and Nutrition Board
ROSE MARIE MARTINEZ, Director, Board on Population Health and Public Health Practice
GERALDINE KENNEDO, Administrative Assistant

FOOD AND NUTRITION BOARD

Independent Report Reviewers

This workshop summary has been reviewed in draft form by individuals chosen for their diverse perspectives and technical expertise, in accordance with procedures approved by the National Research Council's Report Review Committee. The purpose of this independent review is to provide candid and critical comments that will assist the institution in making its published summary as sound as possible and to ensure that the summary meets institutional standards for objectivity, evidence, and responsiveness to the study charge. The review comments and draft manuscript remain confidential to protect the integrity of the deliberative process. We wish to thank the following individuals for their review of this summary:

I-MIN LEE, Harvard Medical School and Harvard School of Public Health, Boston, MA
JAMES R. MORROW, JR., Department of Kinesiology, Health Promotion, and Recreation, University of North Texas, Denton
MIRIAM E. NELSON, John Hancock Center for Physical Activity and Nutrition, The Gerald J. and Dorothy R. Friedman School of Nutrition Science and Policy, Tufts University, Boston, MA
KENNETH E. POWELL, Public Health Consultant, Atlanta, GA

Although the reviewers listed above have provided many constructive comments and suggestions, they did not see the summary before its release. The review of this summary was overseen by **HUGH H. TILSON,** University of North Carolina, who was appointed by the

Institute of Medicine. He was responsible for making certain that an independent examination of this summary was carried out in accordance with institutional procedures and that all review comments were carefully considered.

Acknowledgments

The collective efforts of many individuals made it possible to plan and conduct the Institute of Medicine (IOM) workshop on the Adequacy of Evidence for Physical Activity Guidelines Development and to prepare this workshop summary within a very short time frame. We are grateful for the assistance of many individuals. RADM Penelope Slade-Royall from the U.S. Department of Health and Human Services, Office of Public Health and Science, Office of Disease Prevention and Health Promotion (DHHS, OPHS, ODPHP) secured DHHS resources to sponsor this effort. CAPT Richard Troiano and Jennifer Tucker from ODPHP, Melissa Johnson from the President's Council on Physical Fitness and Sports, and Harold W. (Bill) Kohl III from the Centers for Disease Control and Prevention provided useful suggestions in planning the workshop. Members of the planning committee (Bill Haskell, Rodney Dishman, Joseph Donnelly, Bruce Jones, and Miriam Nelson) provided invaluable input in planning the workshop agenda and speakers and provided feedback on specific issues related to the written summaries of the presentations. The session speakers prepared insightful presentations, and the discussants were instrumental in identifying areas of controversy and providing supplementary information. The moderators kept the presenters and discussants on task and synthesized the evidence presented in the closing session.

We also appreciate the oversight for the National Academies' review process provided by Bronwyn Schrecker Jamrock and Clyde Behney, skillful copyediting by Mark Goodin, formatting by Judy Estep, manuscript preparation and reference checks conducted by Shannon Wisham, and the careful review and oversight of the report production process by Lara Andersen, Sally Stanfield, and others at the National

Academies Press. We also thank Linda Meyers, Director of the Food and Nutrition Board; Rose Marie Martinez, Director of the Board on Population Health and Public Health Practice; Anton Bandy, Financial Associate; and Shannon Wisham, Research Associate, for assistance. Special thanks are extended to Geraldine Kennedo, Administrative Assistant, for her skillful logistical coordination of the workshop.

Carol West Suitor and Vivica I. Kraak, Rapporteurs

Contents

APPENDIXES

Overview

Is there a sufficient evidence base for the U.S. Department of Health and Human Services (DHHS) to develop a comprehensive set of physical activity guidelines for Americans? To address this question, the Food and Nutrition Board and the Board on Population Health and Public Health Practice, both of the Institute of Medicine (IOM), collaboratively planned the Workshop on the Adequacy of Evidence for Physical Activity Guidelines Development. The workshop, which was sponsored by DHHS, was held in Washington, DC, on October 23–24, 2006.

Thirty expert research scientists and physical activity practitioners from government and academia gave formal presentations during the workshop. The invited workshop moderators, speakers, and discussants were asked to consider the available evidence related to physical activity and the general population, as well as special population subgroups including children and adolescents, pregnant and postpartum women, older adults, and persons with disabilities. Additionally, presenters were asked to consider specific issues of relevance in assessing the quality and breadth of the available evidence. However, presenters were asked not to conduct a systematic review of the evidence for a particular population or topic, and they were advised not to propose physical activity guidelines at the workshop.

The planning committee's role was limited to planning the workshop, and the workshop summary has been prepared by the workshop rapporteurs as a factual summary of what occurred at the workshop.

THE WORKSHOP

The chair of the planning group, Dr. William L. Haskell, served as the overall moderator for the workshop. He was assisted by seven colleagues who moderated the presentations and discussions for six plenary sessions. After an overview of the purpose and structure of the workshop, expert panels addressed the amount and strength of the evidence relating physical activity to health promotion and chronic disease prevention, obesity and weight management, and risks of harm. Later in the program, special consideration was given to children and youth, pregnant and postpartum women, older adults, and persons with disabilities and chronic health conditions. Periodically, scheduled discussants provided supplementary information on each major topic. During each group discussion, members of the audience provided additional evidence, raised questions, and suggested additional points for consideration by DHHS. At the end of the workshop, moderators summarized the evidence related to the major topics covered and identified a number of issues that would need to be considered if DHHS decides to develop evidence-informed physical activity guidelines for Americans.

This report is a summary of the workshop presentations and discussions. Appendix A provides the workshop agenda, Appendix B contains the biographical sketches of the presenters, and Appendix C lists the workshop participants. For convenience, Appendix D identifies acronyms and abbreviations, and Appendix E provides a glossary of selected terms. The transcripts and slides used during presentations served as the basis for the summary, but some of the content has been rearranged for greater clarity. None of the statements made in this workshop summary represents conclusions, recommendations, or group consensus. Two terms used throughout the summary merit special attention. *Physical activity* refers to body movement that is produced by the contraction of skeletal muscle and that substantially increases energy expenditure. *Exercise* often refers to planned, structured, and repetitive body movement to improve or maintain one or more components of physical fitness. In some cases, these two terms are used interchangeably.

As indicated in Chapter 8, which covers the closing session, a sizable body of literature was identified that documents a wide variety of benefits of physical activity for all the population groups examined. For each outcome, the strength of the evidence and the amount of evidence varies depending on the topic. Overall, the body of evidence includes large and small randomized controlled trials, meta-analyses and systematic reviews, prospective observational studies, consecutive case series, case–control studies, genetic studies, and studies of biological mechanisms. In addition, considerable evidence addresses the risks associated with physical activity, ways to reduce the risks, and considerations in weighing the risks against the benefits. Although the final chapter summarizes information from the closing session on the amount and strength of the available evidence, this information does not represent conclusions or recommendations at this workshop.

1

Introductory Session

This workshop brought together expert research scientists and physical activity practitioners from academia and government to explore the adequacy of evidence for physical activity guidelines development. This activity was a quick response to a request made by the U.S. Department of Health and Human Services (DHHS) to the Institute of Medicine (IOM) to organize a 2-day workshop to determine whether sufficient evidence exists for DHHS to proceed in a systematic way to develop a comprehensive set of physical activity guidelines for Americans.

According to RADM Penelope Slade Royall, one of the greatest challenges at DHHS is leading the American public to be more physically active. Over the past 30 years, the federal government and many organizations have issued physical activity recommendations. Although the various recommendations illustrate the scientific consensus on the health benefits of physical activity, they differ from each other with regard to particular details: How much physical activity? What type of activity? For whom and how often? Scientific advances may make it possible to develop comprehensive guidance targeted to children, youth, adults, and older adults. RADM Royall indicated that DHHS planned to use the information presented at this IOM workshop to determine whether to move forward on developing comprehensive physical activity guidelines for Americans.

WORKSHOP GOALS

Presenter: William L. Haskell

The purpose of the workshop was twofold: (1) examine the available data that link physical activity to health, giving special emphasis on the nature and strength of the evidence; and (2) identify areas in which research is needed to develop *evidence-informed* physical activity guidelines with confidence. The term *evidence-informed* refers to the accumulation of data from a wide variety of research designs and clinical experiences to reach a solid conclusion. Figure 1-1 illustrates the nature of evidence-informed guidelines for public health policy.

Evidence-informed physical activity guidelines could be substantially more comprehensive than the physical activity guidelines contained in the Dietary Guidelines for Americans 2005 (DHHS and USDA, 2005), but they also would need to coordinate with those guidelines. This workshop was planned to address evidence related to a broad range of health outcomes (both benefits and risks) and many subpopulations, including children and youth, adults, pregnant and postpartum women, older persons, and persons with disabilities.

The presenters were cautioned to avoid making recommendations for physical activity guidelines. Rather, they were asked to provide scientific evidence that DHHS could use to make a decision regarding whether to move forward on developing guidelines and, if the decision was positive, that would provide a useful starting point for a future expert panel in developing physical activity guidelines for Americans. Thus each participant was asked to provide a list of relevant scientific references and other supporting materials for their presentations. References related specifically to the presentations are listed at the end of each chapter. Additional references have been forwarded to DHHS staff in the Office of Disease Prevention and Health Promotion.

Dr. Haskell provided an example of the type of evidence that would be considered if U.S. Food and Drug Administration (FDA) approval was required before physical activity could be promoted as a "medicine" or therapy. Such approval would require evidence on the following:

- *Efficacy.* Does physical activity cause a specific health benefit as demonstrated by adequately designed clinical trials?

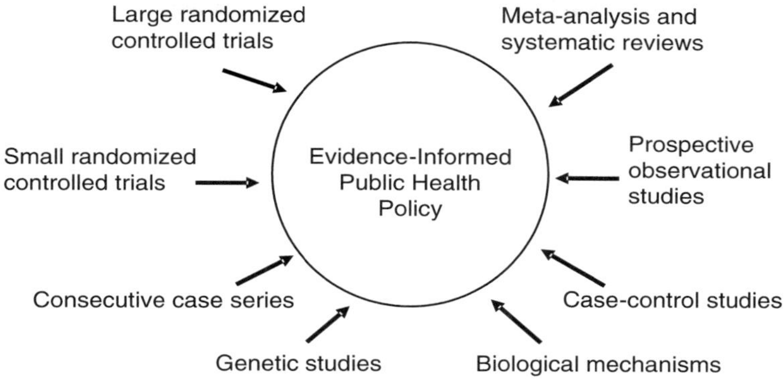

FIGURE 1-1 Research used to support evidence-informed public health policy.
SOURCE: Haskell (2006).

- *Effectiveness.* Is the specified benefit obtained by a reasonable percentage of the persons who undertake the prescribed regimen or activity? Who will be a responder, and who will be a nonresponder?
- *Dose.* What dose of physical activity provides a meaningful benefit for a specific condition? The prescribed dose needs to be defined in terms of type, intensity, frequency, and duration or amount.
- *Mechanisms of action.* What changes in structure or function caused by the physical activity are responsible for the specific health benefit? In a therapy such as physical activity, there may be multiple mechanisms for a single health benefit.
- *Potential adverse events.* What are the medical risks associated with the prescribed dose of physical activity? What are the medical contraindications for the prescribed activity, and what adjustments in dose are needed for specific populations to maximize the benefits and reduce adverse events?

Data that support each of these areas could provide the scientific evidence base to develop broad national physical activity guidelines for Americans.

STATE OF THE NATION RELATIVE TO PHYSICAL ACTIVITY RECOMMENDATIONS FOR AMERICANS

Presenter: Russell R. Pate

History of Physical Activity Guidelines

The first physical activity guidelines in the United States were developed in 1975. Box 1-1 lists the American College of Sports Medicine's (ACSM's) recommended doses of aerobic physical activity and lists key physical activity guidance statements that have been published since 1994. Guidelines for children are not separated from those for adults because some statements were intended to address the physical activity needs of all Americans.

BOX 1-1
Chronological Listing of Physical Activity Guidelines Published from 1975 Through 2005

Recommended Dose of Aerobic Physical Activity, American College of Sports Medicine, 1975 to 2000

For Cardiorespiratory Fitness

1975: 3 to 5 days/week for 20 to 45 minutes/day at 70 to 90 percent of heart rate range (the difference between resting and maximal heart rate, typically 70 to 200 beats per minute in a young adult).

1980 and 1986: 3 to 5 days/week for 15 to 60 minutes/day at 70 to 85 percent of heart rate range.

1991: lower level of intensity reduced to 60 percent of heart rate range.

1995: lower level of intensity reduced to 50 percent of heart rate range and lower level of duration changed to 20 minutes/day.

For Health

2000: 7 days/week for more than 20 minutes/day at 40 to 85 percent of heart rate range.

ACSM's guidance was a gradual decrease in the lower level of the recommended intensity–from quite an intense level of exercise (70 percent of a person's heart rate range in 1975 to 40 percent of a person's heart rate range beginning in 1991).

ACSM (1975, 1980, 1986, 1991, 1995, 2000)

BOX 1-1 Continued

San Diego Consensus Physical Activity Guidelines for Adolescents

- All adolescents should be physically active daily, or nearly every day, as part of play, games, sports, transportation, recreation, physical education, or physical exercise, in the context of family, school, and community activities.
- Adolescents should engage in three or more sessions per week of activities that last 20 minutes or more at a time and that require moderate to vigorous levels of exertion.

Sallis and Patrick (1994)

Physical Activity and Public Health: A Recommendation from the Centers for Disease Control and Prevention and the American College of Sports Medicine

Every U.S. adult should accumulate 30 minutes or more of moderate-intensity physical activity on most, and preferably all days of the week.

Pate et al. (1995)

Physical Activity and Health: A Report from the Surgeon General

- People of all ages should accumulate at least 30 minutes of physical activity of moderate intensity on most if not all days of the week.
- Activity leading to an increase in daily expenditure of approximately 150 kilocalories/day (equivalent to approximately 1,000 kilocalories/week) is associated with substantial health benefits and the activity does not need to be vigorous to achieve benefit.

DHHS (1996)

NIH Consensus Development Panel on Physical Activity and Cardiovascular Health

All Americans should engage in regular physical activity at a level appropriate to their capacity, need, and interest. Children and adults alike should set a goal of accumulating at least 30 minutes of moderate-intensity physical activity on most, and preferably all days of the week.

NIH (1995, 1996)

Health Education Authority Recommendations

- All children and youth should participate in physical activity that is of at least moderate intensity for an average of one hour per day. While young people should be physically active nearly every day, the amount of physical activity can appropriately vary from day to day in type, setting, intensity, duration, and amount.
- All children and youth should participate at least twice per week in physical activities that enhance and maintain strength in the musculature of the trunk and upper arm girdle.

Cavill et al. (2001)

Continued

BOX 1-1 Continued

Institute of Medicine Dietary Reference Intakes
In addition to the activities identified with a sedentary lifestyle, an average of 60 minutes of daily moderate-intensity physical activity or shorter periods of more vigorous exertion was associated with a normal BMI and therefore is recommended for normal-weight individuals.

IOM (2002/2005)

Dietary Guidelines for Americans 2005
Adults
- To reduce the risk of chronic disease in adulthood, engage in at least 30 minutes of moderate intensity physical activity.
- To help manage body weight and prevent gradual unhealthy weight gain in adulthood, engage in approximately 60 minutes of moderate-to-vigorous intensity activity.

Children and Adolescents
- At least 60 minutes of moderate to vigorous physical activity is recommended on most days to maintain good health and fitness and for healthy weight during growth. Increasing physical activity can lower the body mass index of overweight children.
- During leisure time, it is advisable for all individuals to limit sedentary behaviors, such as television watching and video viewing, and replace them with activities that require more movement.

DHHS and USDA (2005)

Evidence-Based Physical Activity for School-Aged Youth
School-aged youth should participate every day in 60 minutes of more of moderate to vigorous physical activity that is enjoyable and developmentally appropriate.

Strong et al. (2005)

National Association for Sports & Physical Education
Guidelines for Toddlers and Preschoolers
- Toddlers should accumulate at least 30 minutes/day and preschoolers should accumulate at least 60 minutes/day of structured physical activity.
- Toddlers and preschoolers should engage in at least 60 minutes and up to several hours per day of daily, unstructured physical activity and should not be sedentary for more than 60 minutes at a time except when sleeping.

NASPE (2006)

Adults

From the early 1970s to the early 1990s, physical activity recommendations for the U.S. population were embodied in an exercise prescription that specified at least 20 minutes/day of probably structured, vigorous (or what would be perceived as vigorous) exercise 3 to 5 days a week (Box 1-1). Exercise physiology research supported the view that activity performed in that way would produce improvements in physical fitness and in some other health parameters. Over that early period, the major change in ACSM's guidance was a gradual decrease in the lower level of the recommended intensity—from quite an intense level of exercise (70 percent of the person's heart rate range[1]) in 1975 to 40 percent of the person's heart rate range beginning in 1991 (ACSM, 1975, 1991, 1995) (Box 1-1).

In 1992, the American Heart Association (AHA) took an important action by declaring that physical inactivity was a major risk factor for cardiovascular diseases (CVD) (AHA, 1992). Many investigators recognized an inconsistency between the recommendation that physical activity should be performed and structured in vigorous ways and the evidence in the epidemiological literature, which suggested that there might be many different ways to produce important health benefits through physical activity.

Subsequently, the Centers for Disease Control and Prevention (CDC) and ACSM developed and jointly released the recommendation that every U.S. adult should accumulate 30 minutes or more of moderate-intensity physical activity on most or preferably all days of the week (Pate et al., 1995). The novel elements in that guideline were its sanctioning of moderate-intensity physical activity and the concept that short bouts of activity could be accumulated by individuals throughout the day. The core guidance provided in *Physical Activity and Health: A Report of the Surgeon General* (DHHS, 1996) and by a National Institutes of Health consensus conference (NIH, 1995; NIH Consensus Development Panel on Physical Activity and Cardiovascular Health, 1996) was essentially the same as the CDC and ACSM recommendation.

Compared with earlier guidelines, one physical activity recommendation that was released by IOM (IOM, 2002/2005) called for a longer duration (60 minutes) of moderate-intensity physical activity daily, in

---

[1]The heart rate range refers to the difference between the resting and maximal heart rate. For a young adult, for example, the heart rate range typically would be about 130 beats per minute (the difference between 70 and 200 beats per minute).

addition to the activities required by a sedentary lifestyle, to prevent weight gain, as well as to accrue additional weight-independent health benefits of physical activity. The recommendations introduced in the Dietary Guidelines for Americans 2005 (DHHS and USDA, 2005) were related but somewhat different from the recommendations in the IOM report. Over the 30 years since the release of the 1975 ACSM exercise recommendation, many people have appeared resistant to accepting the newer physical activity recommendations.

Children and Youth

The effort to develop physical activity guidelines specifically for young people began in the mid-1990s (Box 1-1). The San Diego Consensus Physical Activity Guidelines for Adolescents (Sallis and Patrick, 1994) and the Health Education Authority Recommendations (Cavill et al., 2001) were based on very limited data. In the publication by Strong and colleagues (2005), an expert panel conducted an extensive systematic literature review on the evidence associating physical activity with health and other outcomes in children and youth. The panel recommended that school-age youth participate in 60 minutes or more of daily moderate to vigorous physical activity that is developmentally appropriate. The guidelines for children and youth that were included in the Dietary Guidelines for Americans 2005 are consistent with Strong et al. (2005). A different expert group convened by the National Association for Sport & Physical Education (NASPE) developed the first physical activity guidelines for toddlers and preschoolers under the age of 5 years (NASPE, 2006) (Box 1-1).

Current Adherence with Existing Guidelines

The Behavioral Risk Factor Surveillance System (BRFSS) is the primary source of data that tracks the extent to which Americans are meeting established physical activity recommendations. The 2001 BRFSS determined the percentages of individuals who, by self-report, engaged either in 30 minutes per day of moderate-intensity activity on 5 or more days per week or in 20 minutes per day of vigorous-intensity activity on 3 or more days per week. The percentage of persons meeting the standard decreases from about 60 percent in the youngest group to less than 40 percent in the oldest group (Macera et al., 2005). Rates of physical activity vary by racial or ethnic background, sex, and age. Similar data are available from the Youth Risk Behavior Surveillance System (YRBSS) (Eaton et al., 2006); however, Dr. Pate questioned how accurately YRBSS estimates the level of physical activity for children and youth.

The application of accelerometry as an objective measure of physical activity is making it possible to track physical activity more accurately than by self-report. Figure 1-2, which is based on accelerometry data, shows the mean number of minutes of daily moderate to vigorous physical activity, counting bouts lasting 10 minutes or more, for groups ranging in age from 6 years to older than 70 years. Clearly, most people are physically active for fewer than 30 minutes/day.

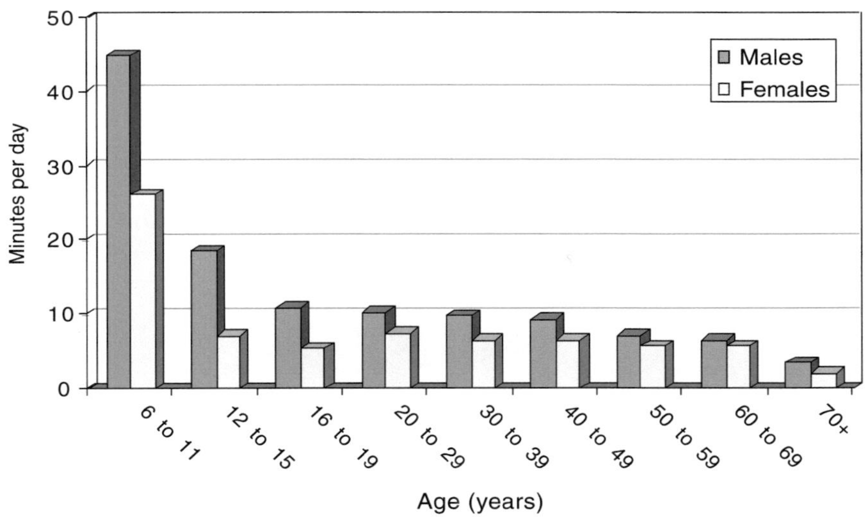

FIGURE 1-2 Mean moderate to vigorous physical activity minutes per day obtained using accelerometry data from the National Health and Nutrition Examination Survey, 2003–2004, and counting modified bouts of at least a 10-minute duration, by age group and sex.
SOURCE: Richard Troiano, Ph.D., U.S. Department of Health and Human Services, Personal communication, October 13, 2006.

Growth of the Knowledge Base Regarding Physical Activity and Health

Dr. Pate used two quick methods to assess the growth of the knowledge base regarding physical activity and health. The first was to note the change in the number of citations of the 1995 CDC and ACSM physical activity recommendations by year. In both 2004 and 2005, the number peaked at 241 citations. The second method was to examine the results of PubMed searches that used the key terms *health and exercise* and *health and physical activity* to identify publications from 1980 through 2005. Figure 1-3 depicts the curvilinear growth in the number of published papers on these topics over the past 25 years.

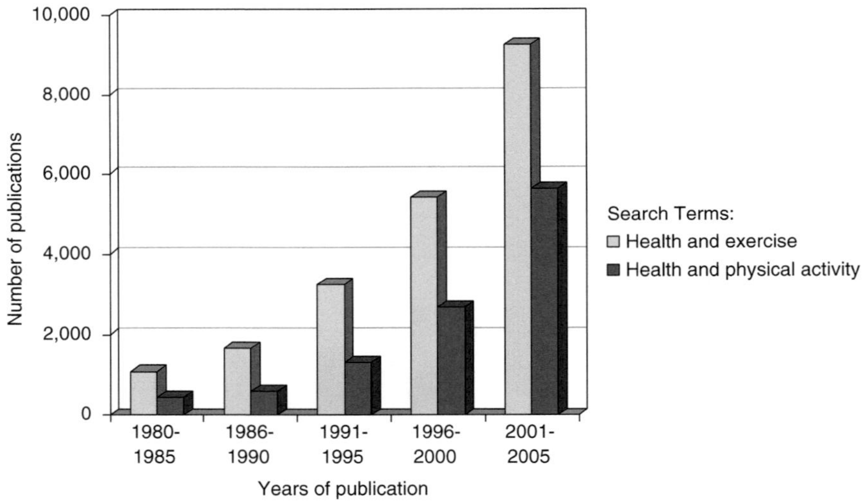

FIGURE 1-3 Increase in publications identified by searching PubMed for *health and exercise* and *health and physical activity* for 5-year intervals from 1980 through 2005.
NOTE: The search was conducted in 2006.
SOURCE: Pate (2006).

Concluding Remarks

Dr. Pate emphasized that we are in a period of developing improved methods for measuring physical activity and that this issue would need to be addressed by an expert group developing physical activity guidelines for Americans. Regardless of the measurement method used, most demographic groups have low adherence to the current physical activity guidelines. Dr. Pate underscored the need for major public health initiatives to promote physical activity. One such initiative would be the development of comprehensive physical activity guidelines for the American public.

REFERENCES

ACSM (American College of Sports Medicine). 1975. *Guidelines for Graded Exercise Testing and Exercise Prescription.* Philadelphia, PA: Lea & Febiger.

ACSM. 1980. *Guidelines for Graded Exercise Testing and Exercise Prescription.* Philadelphia, PA: Lea & Febiger.

ACSM. 1986. *Guidelines for Graded Exercise Testing and Exercise Prescription.* Philadelphia, PA: Lea & Febiger.

ACSM. 1991. *Guidelines for Graded Exercise Testing and Exercise Prescription.* Philadelphia, PA: Lea & Febiger.

ACSM. 1995. *Guidelines for Graded Exercise Testing and Exercise Prescription.* Philadelphia, PA: Lea & Febiger.

ACSM. 2000. *Guidelines for Graded Exercise Testing and Exercise Prescription.* Philadelphia, PA: Lea & Febiger.

AHA (American Heart Association). 1992. Statement on exercise. Benefits and recommendations for physical activity programs for all Americans: A statement for health professionals by the Committee on Exercise and Cardiac Rehabilitation of the Council on Clinical Cardiology, American Heart Association. *Circulation* 86(1):340–344.

Cavill N, Biddle S, Sallis JF. 2001. Health enhancing physical activity for young people: Statement of the United Kingdom Expert Consensus Conference. *Ped Exerc Sci* 13:12–25.

DHHS (U.S. Department of Health and Human Services). 1996. *Physical Activity and Health: A Report of the Surgeon General.* Office of the Surgeon General, Atlanta, GA: Centers for Disease Control and Prevention, National Center for Chronic Disease Prevention and Health Promotion. [Online]. Available: http://www.cdc.gov/nccdphp/sgr/pdf/sgrfull.pdf [accessed November 14, 2006].

DHHS and USDA (U.S. Department of Agriculture). 2005. *Dietary Guidelines for Americans 2005*. [Online]. Available: http://www.healthierus.gov/dietary guidelines [accessed November 14, 2006].

Eaton DK, Kann L, Kinchen S, Ross J, Hawkins J, Harris WA, Lowry R, McManus T, Chyen D, Shanklin S, Lim C, Grunbaum JA, Wechsler H. 2006. Youth risk behavior surveillance—United States, 2005. *MMWR* 55(5):1–108. [Online]. Available: http://www.cdc.gov/mmwr/PDF/SS/SS5505.pdf [accessed November 14, 2006].

Haskell WL. 2006. *Research to Support Evidence-Informed Public Health Policy. Opening Session.* Workshop Purpose and Scope. Presentation at the Institute of Medicine Workshop on Physical Activity Guidelines Development. Washington, DC. October 23.

IOM (Institute of Medicine). 2002/2005. *Dietary Reference Intakes: Energy, Carbohydrates, Fiber, Fat, Fatty Acids, Cholesterol, Protein, and Amino Acids*. Washington, DC: The National Academies Press.

Macera CA, Ham SA, Yore MM, Jones DA, Ainsworth BE, Kimsey CD, Kohl HW. 2005. Prevalence of physical activity in the United States: Behavioral Risk Factor Surveillance System, 2001. *Prev Chronic Dis* 2(2):A17.

NASPE (National Association for Sport & Physical Education) and AHA (American Heart Association). 2006. *2006 Shape of the Nation Report.* [Online]. Available: http://www.aahperd.org/naspe/ShapeOfTheNation/ [accessed November 14, 2006].

NIH (National Institutes of Health). 1995. Consensus development conference statement on physical activity and cardiovascular health. *J Am Med Assoc* 13(3):1–33.

NIH Consensus Development Panel on Physical Activity and Cardiovascular Health. 1996. Physical activity and cardiovascular health. *J Am Med Assoc* 276(3):241–246.

Pate RR. 2006. *The Evolution of Public Health Guidelines on Physical Activity.* Presentation at the Institute of Medicine Workshop on Physical Activity Guidelines Development. Washington, DC. October 23.

Pate RR, Pratt M, Blair SN, Haskell WL, Macera CA, Bouchard C, Buchner D, Ettinger W, Heath GW, King AC, Kriska A, Leon AS, Marcus BH, Morris J, Paffenbarger RS Jr, Patrick K, Pollock ML, Rippe JM, Sallis J, Wilmore JH. 1995. Physical activity and public health. A recommendation from the Centers for Disease Control and Prevention and the American College of Sports Medicine. *J Am Med Assoc* 273(5):402–407.

Sallis JF, Patrick K. 1994. Physical activity guidelines for adolescents: Consensus statement. *Ped Exerc Sci* 6:302–314.

Strong WB, Malina RM, Blimkie CJ, Daniels SR, Dishman RK, Gutin B, Hergenroeder AC, Must A, Nixon PA, Pivarnik JM, Rowland T, Trost S, Trudeau F. 2005. Evidence based physical activity for school-age youth. *J Pediatr* 146(6):732–737.

2

Physical Activity, Health Promotion, and Chronic Disease Prevention

The scope of effects of physical activity in health promotion and chronic disease prevention is broad, and the workshop devoted two sessions to the topic as it relates to the general population. This chapter addresses four major topics:

- Cardiovascular disease (CVD), all-cause mortality, and cancer
- Bone, joint, and muscle health and performance
- Mental and neurological health
- Diabetes and other metabolic disorders

Brief coverage of mechanisms of action in diabetes and of physical activity and cognition appears under the discussion section, followed by points raised by participants during the group discussion.

CARDIOVASCULAR DISEASE, ALL-CAUSE MORTALITY, AND CANCER

Presenter: Steven N. Blair

Dr. Blair's presentation began with a historical overview of the topic and the identification of exposure assessment issues, followed by a discussion of physical activity and the relationships among CVD, all-cause mortality, and cancer. As the volume of evidence is very large and time was limited, Dr. Blair selected data pertaining to different populations to illustrate these relationships.

Background

Historical Overview

Although Hippocrates and Galen recognized the benefits of physical activity, the beginning of exercise science occurred in the twentieth century. In the early 1920s, August Krogh and A.V. Hill won separate Nobel Prizes in physiology and medicine for work related to physical activity. A study of London transport workers (Morris et al., 1953) showed much lower rates of coronary occlusion and of death from heart attack among the physically active conductors than among the sedentary drivers. Based on these results, Morris and colleagues formulated the hypothesis that vigorous physical activity helps protect against coronary heart disease (CHD). A study of the relationship of physical activity at work to CHD deaths among longshoremen (Paffenbarger and Hale, 1975) provided further strong evidence of the benefits of physical activity.

Exposure Assessment Issues

Self-reported questionnaires have provided valuable evidence of relationships between physical activity and disease outcomes. Nonetheless, some of them have led to a large amount of misclassification. Misclassification, in turn, has led to an underestimation of the observed effect. The objective assessment of physical activity levels, such as the use of accelerometers or specific fitness tests, is expected to provide stronger evidence of the effects of physical activity or inactivity on various health outcomes.

Physical Activity, Fitness, and Cardiovascular Disease

Figure 2-1 illustrates the results obtained from a study of CVD death rates for women and men by fitness category (obtained using an objective test of fitness). Steep inverse gradients occur across the fitness categories. Especially notable is the very large difference in CVD death rates between the low fit and the moderately fit group. That is, one need only achieve the moderately fit category to derive considerable benefit.

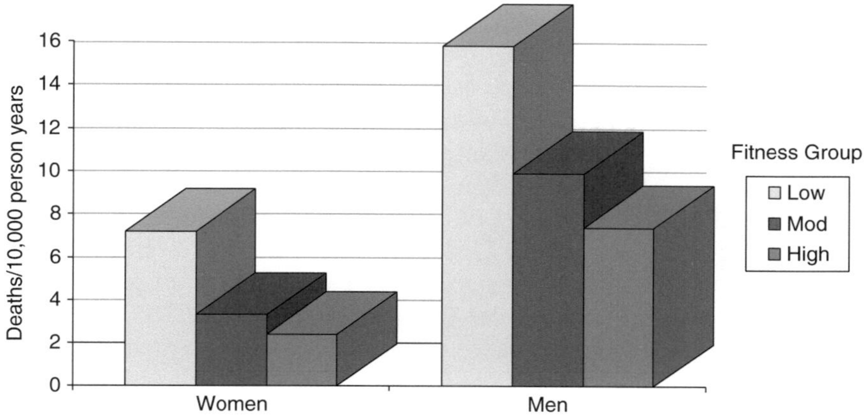

FIGURE 2-1 Cardiovascular death rates by fitness groups and sex. Death rates are adjusted for age, examination year, and other risk factors. The Aerobic Center Longitudinal Study (ACLS) objective test of fitness was used to classify fitness groups.
SOURCE: Blair et al. (1996). Reprinted, with permission, from *JAMA* 276(3):205–210. Copyright ©1996 American Medical Association.

The measurement of inactivity or sedentary behavior may be another useful approach to examining the relationship of physical activity to CVD. For example, Manson and colleagues (2002) showed an increase in the multivariate-adjusted relative risk of CVD with an increase in the number of hours per day spent sitting.

Work by Hambrecht and colleagues (2004) shows that, among individuals with documented coronary artery disease, the group randomly assigned to exercise (20 minutes per day on a cycle ergometer and a 60-minute group aerobic exercise class once per week) had greater event-free survival and exercise capacity than the group assigned to standard treatment and angioplasty.

Unpublished data from the Aerobics Center Longitudinal Study (LaMonte et al., 2005b) show that for both men and women, a greater fitness level is associated with decreasing rates of CVD deaths, CHD events, or CHD deaths. Fitness was assessed by a maximal exercise test on a treadmill and was categorized by the highest level of metabolic equivalent (MET) expenditure. In a multivariate analysis, the reduction of risk per MET was approximately 10 to 15 percent for the various end points in both women and men.

A very recent report from the Nurse's Health Study (Whang et al., 2006), using self-reported data, shows a substantial decrease in the age-adjusted hazard ratio for sudden cardiac death among women who spend more than 3.9 hours per week in moderate to vigorous physical activity. This is one of the first reports to show a relationship between physical activity and a lower risk of sudden cardiac death in women. Evidence is accumulating that coronary artery calcium is an indicator of subclinical CHD among men and women (LaMonte et al., 2005c). A study of 710 asymptomatic men with a coronary artery calcium score of greater than 100 found a very large reduction in the relative risk of CHD events for those having an exercise tolerance of 10 or more METS (Lamonte et al., 2006).

Barlow and colleagues (2006) reported on the risk of incident hypertension among healthy women by fitness group. After adjusting for age and other relevant factors, the risk of developing hypertension was markedly decreased for women in the moderate fitness group and even further decreased for women in the high fitness group. Earlier work had demonstrated this relationship among men.

All-Cause Mortality

Physical activity has been associated with a decreased risk of death in various population groups. A prospective study of 17,265 men and 13,375 women ages 20–93 years in Copenhagen found a substantial decrease in the risk of death among those who spent 3 hours per week commuting to work by bicycle compared to those who did not commute by bicycle (Andersen et al., 2000). Among the men and women ages 60 years and older, the multivariate-adjusted relative risk for all-cause mortality decreased substantially by fitness level. Among men, the death rate for those ages 80 years or older in the high fitness group was lower than that for the least fit men ages 60 to 69 years (Blair and Wei, 2000).

Among men, the relative risk for all-cause and CVD mortality is consistently lower for the fit when compared to the unfit across body fat categories (Lee et al., 1999). In other words, being moderately fit is associated with a substantially greater chance of survival even among those with 25 percent of their body weight as fat. Similarly, among men with metabolic syndrome, those in the moderate and high cardiorespiratory fitness groups have increasingly lower all-cause mortality than do the less fit men (Katzmarzyk et al., 2004).

The length of time required to complete a 400-meter walk—a different kind of objective fitness test—is a predictor of mortality, CVD, and mobility disability among women and men ages 70 to 79 years at baseline (Newman et al., 2006). Differences in energy expenditure measured with doubly labeled water methods produce similar results (Manini et al., 2006).

Measuring physical activity level by accelerometer, Garg and colleagues (2006) found than men and women with peripheral artery disease had decreasing multivariate-adjusted rates of all-cause mortality with increasing levels of physical activity.

Findings in a paper by Erikssen and colleagues (1998) are consistent with those of a number of other papers reporting decreasing multivariate-adjusted relative risk of mortality with improvements in cardiorespiratory fitness. Changing one's fitness level affects mortality risk. These observations strengthen the causal inference for the effect of physical activity in lowering the risk of death.

Physical Activity, Fitness, and Cancer

The body of literature on physical activity and cancer is smaller than that discussed above, but it is growing. Three examples of relevant study results follow:

- Women diagnosed with breast cancer had a lower multivariate-adjusted relative risk of death and of recurrence if they obtained at least 3 MET-hours of activity per week than if they had a lower exercise level (Holmes et al., 2005).
- In a study of men with gastric cancer in Japan, the least fit one-fourth of the group (tested by cycle odometer) were much more likely to die of gastric cancer than was the more fit group (Sawada et. al., 2003).
- Farrell and colleagues (2006) report that the inverse association of cardiorespiratory fitness with cancer mortality remains after adjustment for the percentage of body fat.

Concluding Remarks

We have and are accumulating a very large amount of evidence on the effects of physical activity and fitness on a variety of health outcomes. For nearly every health outcome examined and in nearly every subgroup of the population, physical activity provides benefits. Dr. Blair expressed the view that there is a sufficient evidence base for understanding the benefits of physical activity and chronic disease prevention, and he suggested that the U.S. Department of Health and Human Services move forward with a process for developing physical activity guidelines for Americans.

BONE, JOINT, AND MUSCLE HEALTH AND PERFORMANCE

Presenter: Wendy M. Kohrt

In addressing the role of physical activity in bone, joint, and muscle health and performance, Dr. Kohrt focused on bone mineral content (BMC)—the amount of mineral at a particular skeletal site, such as the femoral neck, lumbar spine, or total body; bone mineral density (BMD)—the value determined by dividing the bone mineral content by the area of a scanned region; osteoporotic fracture risk, osteoarthritis, and muscle mass and function (quality). Performance related to mobility and functional abilities was covered by Dr. Fielding. (See Chapter 6, Physical Activity and Special Considerations for Older Adults.)

Bone Health

Many studies show positive effects of either a physically active lifestyle or exercise interventions on intermediate markers of bone health, such as BMC and BMD. The evidence regarding the effects of physical activity on the risk of osteoporosis comes from randomized controlled trials of exercise intervention, meta-analyses of those trials, trials of the effects of immobilization and unloading, observational studies, and others. The intensity of the exercise appears to be a key determinant of the osteogenic response.

Intervention Studies

A meta-analysis from the Cochrane database involved 18 exercise intervention trials involving more than 1,400 postmenopausal women (Bonaiuti et al., 2002). Results were reported as mean differences between the exercise and the control groups and the change in BMD in percentile units. Any type of exercise showed a benefit (approximately a 1.8 percent increase on lumbar spine BMD, and walking benefited both spine and hip BMD).

A slightly larger meta-analysis by Wallace and Cumming (2000) found that impact exercise had significant benefits among postmenopausal women on both lumbar spine and femoral neck BMD. Nonimpact exercise (primarily weight lifting) benefited lumbar spine BMD in postmenopausal women. Essentially the same results were found in studies involving premenopausal women. Randomized controlled trials of exercise interventions in men and children generally have shown benefits on BMD, but they have not yet been included in meta-analyses.

Observational Studies

Physical activity and risk of fracture The question remains about whether an increase in BMD—along with balance, mobility, and muscle strength—decreases the risk of fractures. No randomized controlled trials are available, but some prospective observational studies provide useful data about physical activity and hip fracture risk. The report by Feskanich et al. (2002) from the Nurses' Health Study of more than 60,000 women serves as a good example. The physical activity data are self-reported. The incidence of hip fracture was collected for a 12-year period. The women with the highest level of activity measured in MET-hours per week had about a 50 percent relative risk reduction in hip fracture. Similarly, as walking time increased, hip fracture risk decreased; those who walked more briskly appeared to gain more benefit. The women who became less active over a 6-year period had a statistically significant increase in risk for hip fracture.

Effects of unloading or reduced loading Extreme conditions of physical inactivity or reduced mechanical loading (such as limb immobilization, bed rest, microgravity) cause rapid and profound bone loss. The likelihood for full recovery of mineral is low. A meta-analysis of the effects of bed rest (Law et al., 1991) suggests that 3 weeks of bed rest doubles the risk for hip fractures during the subsequent 10 years. A study by van der Poest et al. (1999) compared the BMD of a person's fractured tibia to that of the healthy tibia for 5 years after the fracture. The 8-week period of unloading subsequent to the fracture resulted in a substantially lower BMD in the injured limb even 5 years after the fracture.

Data Limitations

Little evidence is available on dose–response with respect to how the type, frequency, duration, and/or intensity of exercise affects bone. Because the duration of follow-up in intervention studies has been quite short, little is known about the extent to which the benefits of the interventions are retained. Bone strength (e.g., resistance to fracture) cannot be measured directly in humans, and there is a paucity of information on the relationship between BMD and bone strength. Therefore, the effects of physical activity on BMD may not accurately reflect the effects on resistance to fracture.

Animal Studies

On the other hand, a study conducted in rats showed that loading causes small changes in BMC and BMD that resulted in very large increases in bone strength (Turner and Robling, 2003), as illustrated in Figure 2-2. Thus evidence in animals suggests that physical activity or mechanical loading probably affects the skeleton in a way that translates into large gains in bone strength.

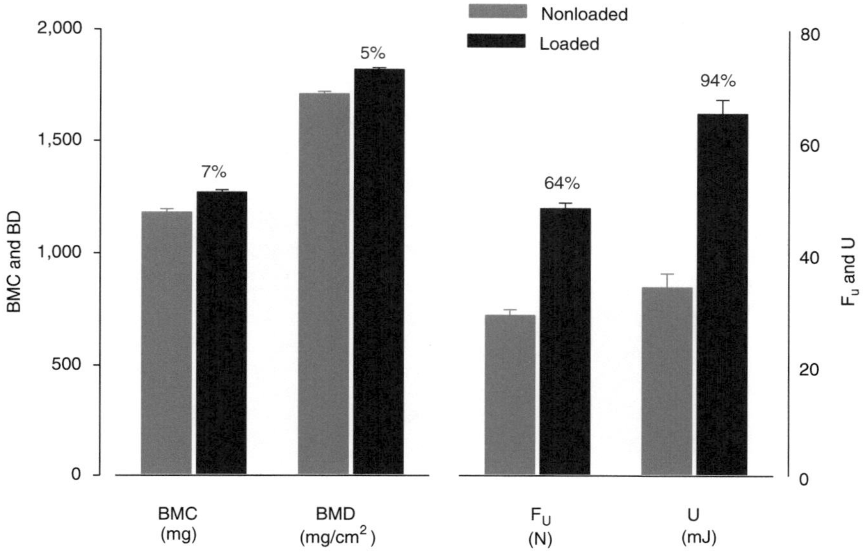

FIGURE 2-2 Effects of mechanical loading on bone mineral content, bone mineral density, ultimate force (the maximum amount of force supported before failure), and energy to fail (the amount of energy absorbed by the bone before failure).
NOTE: BMC = bone mineral content, BMD = bone mineral density, F_U = ultimate force, N = newtons, U = energy to fail, and mJ = millijoules.
SOURCE: Adapted from Turner and Robling (2003). Reprinted with permission from *Exerc Sport Sci Rev.*

Possible Mechanisms by Which Physical Activity Reduces Risk for Osteoporotic Fracture

Four mechanisms may explain the beneficial effects of physical activity in reducing the risk of osteoporotic fracture. Physical activity

1. Increases bone mineral accrual during maturation
2. Attenuates the rate of bone mineral loss during aging
3. Enhances bone strength
4. Reduces the risk of falls by improving muscle strength, flexibility, coordination, and balance

Summary of Effects of Physical Activity on Bone

Moderate to strong evidence indicates that physical activity plays an important role in optimizing bone health during the developmental years; but the long-term effects of benefit are not well known, and dose–response information is lacking. In adulthood, moderate to strong evidence from observational studies suggests that physical activity helps prevent fractures, and randomized controlled trials indicate benefits of physical activity on such useful biomarkers as BMD. The effects of extreme disuse are very deleterious. Dose–response data are lacking.

Joint Health

Very little information is available about the pathogenesis of osteoarthritis (OA) and about a role for physical activity in the primary prevention of the disease. Scant evidence is available for a direct relation of physical activity (especially vigorous activity) and articular volume in children (Jones et al., 2003). Systematic reviews, however, indicate that exercise has benefits in the management of OA. Roddy et al. (2005) examined the evidence base for the role of exercise in the management of hip and knee OA and differentiated research-based evidence from expert opinion. Their literature base included 57 intervention trials of exercise for knee OA, 9 intervention trials of exercise for hip OA, and 3 systematic reviews of exercise for knee or hip OA. When they summarized the evidence, they rated it to be very high for the exercise benefits for people with knee OA. In particular, after pooling all the trials and minimizing the variability, the effect sizes range from 0.3 to 0.5 for the effect of exercise on pain. In contrast, they found very little evidence to support a benefit for individuals with hip OA. The amount of evidence also was very low for the type of exercise to recommend, contraindications for exercise, the relationship of exercise to the progression of the OA, and several other propositions. As with bone health, dose–response data are lacking.

Muscle Health

In contrast with bone health and joint health, muscle health is not directly linked with a chronic disease. A few chronic diseases, however, are associated with low muscle mass or impaired muscle function. These include osteoporosis, in which there is a direct association between muscle mass and bone mass; type 2 diabetes mellitus, in which the muscle is resistant to insulin-mediated glucose uptake; and congestive heart failure (CHF), in which there is skeletal muscle mitochondrial dysfunction. The abnormal muscle in CHF may be a result rather than a cause of the disease, whereas low muscle mass and insulin resistance in muscle may be contributing factors to the etiology of osteoporosis and type 2 diabetes mellitus, respectively.

Physical Activity and Muscle Mass

A wealth of evidence indicates that high-intensity resistance exercise induces muscle hypertrophy and that this adaptive response is retained into very old age. Aerobic exercise has little or no anabolic effect on muscle, although disuse causes muscle atrophy. Aerobic fitness does not appear to have any impact on fat-free mass, whereas strength training enhances muscle mass and strength. Using fat-free mass as a surrogate for muscle mass, Holloszy and Kohrt (1995) showed that fat-free mass is preserved until approximately the age of 50 years. Thereafter, a decline occurs, which becomes steeper with advancing age. Combining those data with data from Hawkins et al. (2001) shows the following: (1) men and women who maintain very vigorous levels of endurance or aerobic activity have fat-free mass levels that are comparable to those of sedentary individuals, and (2) the trajectory of change in fat-free mass over time appears to be quite similar in athletes and sedentary individuals. Similarly, Kyle et al. (2004) showed that fat-free mass, estimated with bioelectrical impedance, is essentially the same in sedentary and physically active men and women.

Physical Activity and Muscle Quality

Dr. Kohrt identified the following characteristics of muscle quality:

- Specific torque (Newton-meters per square centimeter)
- Fatigue resistance
- Metabolic function (e.g., insulin resistance)
- Inflammatory state

All four of these factors respond favorably to exercise intervention. In one small study (Arciero et al., 1999), two groups of middle-aged or older individuals with either impaired glucose tolerance or mild type 2 diabetes were treated for 10 days, either with exercise (energy expenditure was about 420 kilocalories/day) or a dietary restriction of approximately 1,100 kilocalories/day. After treatment, both groups disposed of more glucose at any insulin concentration—that is, their muscles were more insulin sensitive. The improvement by the exercise group, however, was significantly better than that of the dietary restriction group.

Westerterp (2000) reviewed evidence that habitual activity level and exercise have little or no effect on the age-related decline in muscle mass but that habitual activity and exercise training clearly have positive effects on muscle function. These effects include muscle fiber type, capillary density, aerobic capacity, and others. Still lacking is evidence of associations of muscle quality with chronic disease risk.

Concluding Remarks

Dr. Kohrt emphasized that there is moderate to strong evidence that physical activity plays an essential role in the maintenance of bone health, although information is lacking on the type and dose of activity required to optimize the benefits. Whether physical activity helps to prevent the development of OA is not known, but there is moderate to strong evidence that physical activity has beneficial effects on pain and disability in people with knee OA. Aerobic exercise has little effect on the preservation of muscle mass but has multiple favorable effects on muscle quality. Conversely, strength training helps to preserve muscle mass with aging.

MENTAL AND NEUROLOGICAL HEALTH

Presenter: Patrick J. O'Connor

Many mental health and neurological concerns may have some association with physical activity. Dr. O'Connor discussed the evidence relating physical activity to the nine disorders that are identified in Figure 2-3.

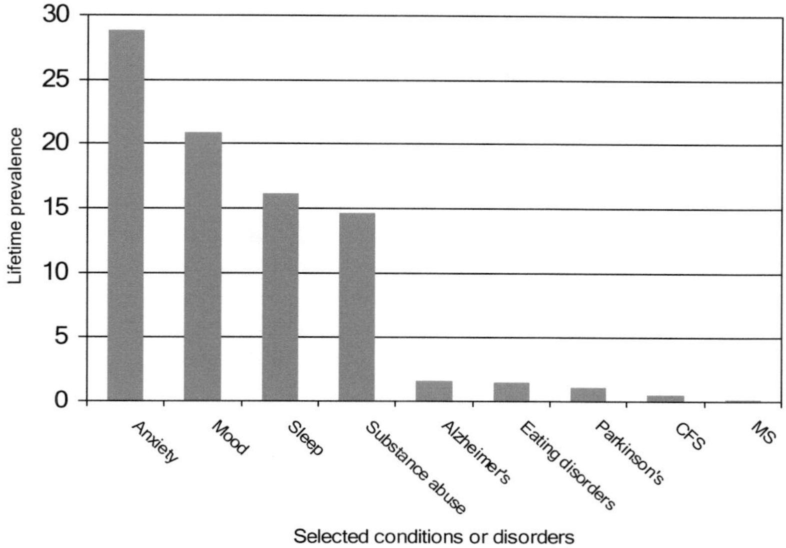

FIGURE 2-3 Estimated lifetime prevalence of selected mental health and neurological disorders.
NOTE: CFS = chronic fatigue syndrome; MS = multiple sclerosis.
SOURCES: de Rijk et al. (1997); Herbert et al. (2001); Jason et al. (1999); Kessler et al. (2006); Morin et al. (2006); Slaughter et al. (2001).

The disorders are shown in decreasing order of the lifetime prevalence of each and are addressed below in that order. Notably, Alzheimer's disease and Parkinson's disease will become more prevalent as the U.S. population ages.

Anxiety

Approximately 50 epidemiological studies address physical activity and anxiety. About 85 percent of these show less severe symptoms of anxiety among physically active adults and youth. For example, the National Comorbidity Study of U.S. adults ages 15–54 years indicates that, after adjusting for a number of variables, persons who are rarely or never physically active tend to report more anxiety disorders than do those who are regularly or occasionally active.

Only one randomized controlled trial (Broocks et al., 1998) addresses the relationship between physical activity and anxiety disorders. The results are shown in Figure 2-4. Notably, when compared with placebo, either 10 weeks of aerobic exercise or treatment with a standard antianxiety medication resulted in significantly better scores on the anxiety scale used.

Animal models provide plausible mechanisms for the benefit of physical activity in reducing anxiety. For example, Dishman (1997) and Fulk et al. (2004) demonstrated anxiety-related changes in behavior and brain biology in rats that had access to a running wheel.

In short, there is a large body of evidence from epidemiological studies of physical activity and anxiety. Physical activity is consistently associated with fewer symptoms of anxiety, the odds of symptoms are reduced by 25 to 50 percent, dose–response is plausible, and a small but increasing body of evidence suggests biologically plausible mechanisms by which physical activity could improve anxiety.

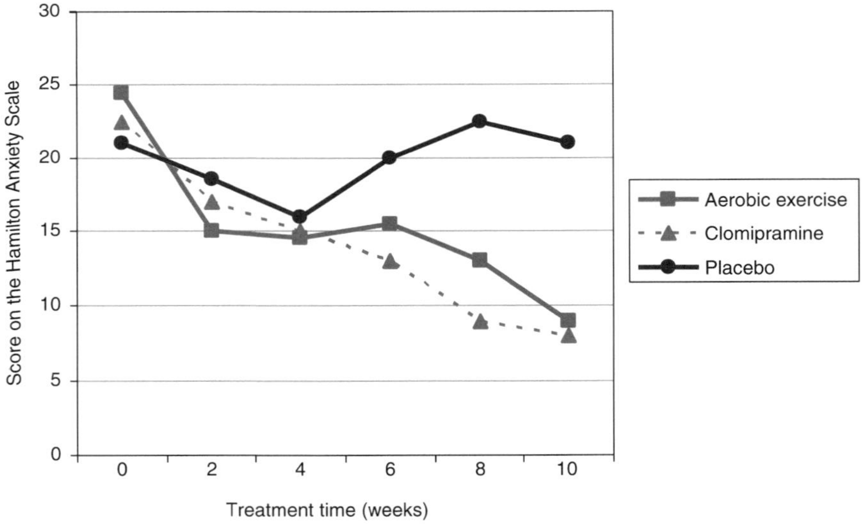

FIGURE 2-4 Comparison of the effects of aerobic exercise training, clomipramine treatments, and placebo on anxiety. Randomized controlled trial of 46 outpatients with panic disorder.
SOURCE: Broocks et al. (1998). Reprinted with permission from the *American Journal of Psychiatry*, Copyright 1996. American Psychiatric Association.

Depression

Nearly 100 studies, most of them quite recent, report on associations between physical activity and depression or symptoms of depression. Approximately 90 percent of the studies show less severe symptoms of depression among physically active adults and youth. The reduction in the odds of symptoms is 30 to 50 percent.

In the Harvard Alumni Study, persons who engaged in more hours of sports or play per week (or who expended more kilocalories by physical activity per week), measured in the 1960s, had a reduced risk for depression during a 23- to 27-year follow-up period (Paffenbarger et al., 1994).

A meta-analysis of 14 randomized controlled trials showed that exercise training reduced symptoms of depression (Lawlor and Hopker, 2001). The standardized mean difference in effect size equaled -1.1, and the confidence interval did not overlap with zero. Many of the trials, however, had methodological limitations. More recently, Dunn and colleagues (2005) conducted a large, rigorously controlled randomized trial that produced results consistent with those of the meta-analysis.

Rodent data show that activity wheel running increases brain-derived neurotropic factor (BDNF) and BDNF mRNA (ribonucleic acid) in the hippocampus and ventral tegmental area (Russo-Neustadt et al., 2000; van Hoomissen et al., 2003). In addition, the running attenuates copulatory deficits in an olfactory bulbectomy model of depression (Chambliss et al., 2004).

In summary, the size of the literature is large, physical activity generally is associated with reduced symptoms of depression, a dose–response is plausible (Dunn et al., 2001), randomized controlled trials (of variable quality) show antidepressant effects of exercise, and evidence suggests biologically plausible mechanisms for the preventive effects of physical activity on anxiety.

Physical Activity and Sleep

Many neurological disorders are associated with poor sleep, and poor sleep itself can have important health-related outcomes. There are approximately 70 sleep disorders, the most studied of which are insomnia and obstructive sleep apnea. One prospective cohort study (Morgan, 2003) examined self-reported insomnia and self-reported physical activity and found that those who reported more activity were less likely to develop insomnia. A cross-sectional study that examined obstructive sleep apnea using polysomnography shows a very large benefit—that less sleep apnea is associated with more reported physical activity (Peppard and Young, 2004).

At least 13 cross-sectional studies show that the chances of having interrupted sleep are lower among persons who are engaged in more physical activity than among persons who have less physical activity or are sedentary (Akerstedt et al., 2002; Kawamoto et al., 2004; Kim et al., 2000; Kravitz et al., 2003; Liu et al., 2000; Morgan, 2003; Nasermoaddeli et al., 2005; Ohayon, 2004; Ohida et al., 2001; Phillips et al., 2000; Sherrill et al., 1998; Surkan et al., 2005; Tynjala et al., 1999). Only two of the 13 trials, Nasermoaddeli et al. (2005) and Surkan et al. (2005), had confidence intervals that overlapped with 1.0, suggesting that the benefit of physical activity is unlikely due to chance.

All the randomized controlled trials show positive effects of exercise training on symptoms of poor sleep (Guilleminault et al., 1995; King et al., 1997, 2002; Littman et al., 2006; Singh et al., 1997, 2005; Tworoger et al., 2003).

Little or no research has been conducted on the biological mechanisms by which exercise could plausibly affect sleep. Indirect evidence suggests that acute bouts of exercise can induce circadian phase shifts (Van Reeth et al., 1994), influence adenosine metabolism (Benington and Heller, 1995), and activate neurological circuits hypothesized to help people feel less anxious and depressed (Youngstedt, 2005). Poor sleep is strongly associated with depression.

In summary, the size of the literature is modest, but it shows that physical activity is consistently associated with both fewer self-reported sleep problems in cross-sectional studies and improved sleep quality in randomized controlled trials. Limited indirect evidence suggests biologically plausible mechanisms by which physical activity could improve sleep or prevent sleep disorders.

Physical Activity and Substance Use or Abuse

Dr. O'Connor was not able to find evidence of associations between physical activity and illicit drug use, and thus did not address this topic in his presentation. Although a large number of epidemiological studies have data on alcohol consumption, generally alcohol use is one of the exposure variables measured rather than an outcome.

Alcohol

A large cross-sectional study by Mukamal et al. (2006) indicates that, on average, those who abstained from alcohol were more sedentary than those who engaged in moderate drinking. Among male runners, the relationship between alcohol consumption and running distance was curvilinear: those who ran less than 16 kilometers per week or more than 64 kilometers per week consumed less alcohol per week.

Cigarette Smoking

Dr. O'Connor highlighted the 15 largest studies that provide data on some type of physical activity and smoking (Baumert et al., 1998; Blair et al., 1985; Boyle et al., 2000; Epstein et al., 1976; Haddock et al., 1998; Hickey et al., 1975; Holme et al., 1981; Pate et al., 1996; Reynolds et al., 2004; Simones et al., 1995; Steptoe et al., 1997; Tretli et al., 1985; Wagner et al., 2003; Ward et al., 2003). The studies ranged in size from nearly 6,000 to more than 128,000 subjects. In general, they showed a negative association between physical activity and smoking.

Ten small to moderate-sized randomized controlled trials examined physical activity and smoking cessation (Ussher, 2005). In general, the effects favor exercise, but none of the studies provides strong evidence that physical activity enhances a smoking cessation program.

Summary

A large literature addresses physical activity related to alcohol consumption and smoking. Several cross-sectional studies suggest nonlinear relationships between physical activity and alcohol consumption. Physical inactivity generally is associated with more smoking in cross-sectional studies. A modest number of randomized controlled trials failed to show that increased physical activity levels lead to significant improvements in smoking cessation. Causal mechanisms have rarely been studied.

Alzheimer's Disease

Ten prospective cohort studies report on the relationship between the level of physical activity and the odds of developing Alzheimer's disease (Abbott et al., 2004; Larson et al., 2006; Lindsay et al., 2002; Podewils et al., 2005; Rovio et al., 2005; Scarmea et al., 2001; Verghese et al., 2003; Wilson et al., 2002a,b; Yoshitake et al., 1995). Although most of the studies show a positive effect, three of the 10 studies (Verghese et al., 2003; Wilson et al., 2002a,b) show a nonsignificant effect; and one of the three studies with nonsignificant findings (Wilson et al., 2002b) had the largest sample size of the 10 cohort studies. Three case–control studies (ranging in size from 60 to 193 cases) report a protective effect of physical activity against Alzheimer's disease (Broe, 1990; Friedland et al., 2001; Kondo et al., 1994).

As reviewed by Heyn et al. (2004), 10 randomized controlled trials have been conducted in older adults with cognitive impairment to examine the effect of exercise on cognitive performance. On average, the effect size (improved cognitive performance) was moderate.

Two studies provide plausible mechanisms for beneficial effects of physical activity in relation to Alzheimer's disease. Transgenic mouse models of Alzheimer's disease show that wheel running decreased extracellular amyloid-β plaques in the frontal cortex and hippocampus (Adlard et al., 2005). A study with a different mouse model found positive effects of physical activity related to up-regulation of hippocampal neurotrophin and brain-derived neurotrophic factor and to increased hippocampal neurogenesis (Wolf et al., 2006).

Dr. O'Connor summarized the small to moderate amount of literature relating physical activity to Alzheimer's disease, emphasizing that physical activity consistently has beneficial effects both on disease development in the observational studies and on cognitive performance in the intervention studies in cognitively impaired older adults. Some evidence supports biologically plausible mechanisms by which physical activity can prevent or attenuate the development of Alzheimer's disease.

Physical Activity and Eating Disorders

There is limited literature on the association between physical activity and eating disorders, and the findings from available studies are controversial and difficult to interpret. There are no randomized controlled trials that have examined the effects of physical activity on eating disorders. This is an area where further research is needed.

Physical Activity and Parkinson's Disease

The size of the literature addressing physical activity and Parkinson's disease is small. Observational studies show mixed evidence that physical activity is associated with a reduced risk of Parkinson's disease (Chen et al., 2005; Logroscino et al., 2006). Of the four case–control studies (Frigerio et al., 2005; Kuopio et al., 1999; Sasco et al., 1992; Tsai et al., 2002), all but Kuopio et al. (1999) show the odds of Parkinson's disease in the active group being lower than those in the less active group. Three small randomized controlled trials (Miyai et al., 2002; Schenkman et al., 1998; Schmitz-Hubsch et al., 2006) all show positive effects of 4 to 10 weeks of exercise on spinal flexibility, movement speed, and disease symptoms when compared to usual care. Data from rodent models of Parkinson's disease suggest biologically plausible mechanisms by which physical activity could prevent or attenuate Parkinson's disease (Cohen et al., 2003; Fisher et al., 2004; Poulton and Muir, 2005; Tillerson et al., 2003). Notably, exercise has been shown to down-regulate the dopamine transporter (Fisher et al. 2004).

Physical Activity and Chronic Fatigue Syndrome

The literature on physical activity and chronic fatigue syndrome is small, and epidemiological studies of this condition rarely have included measures of physical activity. Five relatively small randomized controlled trials all show a positive effect of exercise training on symptoms of chronic fatigue syndrome (Fulcher and White, 1997; Moss-Morris et al., 2005; Powell et al., 2001; Wallman et al., 2004; Weardon et al., 1998). In a review of randomized controlled trials of groups of medical patients and other adults, 70 trials show that exercise training consistently reduces symptoms of fatigue (Puetz et al., 2006).

Physical Activity and Multiple Sclerosis

The literature on physical activity and multiple sclerosis is very small: one cross-sectional study (Stuifbergen et al., 2006), one 5-year prospective cohort study (Stuifbergen et al., 2006), no case-control studies, eight randomized controlled trials (Mostert and Kesslering, 2002; Oken et al., 2004; Petajan et al., 1996; Romberg et al., 2004, 2005; Solari et al., 1999; van den Berg et al., 2006; Wiles et al., 2001), and no studies of causal mechanisms. Most of the studies have few subjects, and the effects observed, although consistently favorable, are small.

Physical Activity and Suicide

The few studies consistently find a small correlation in the direction of a protective effect of sports participation among youth on suicide ideation and attempt (Oler et al., 1994; Page et al., 1998; Tomori and Zalar, 2000; Unger, 1997), but the association is not consistent for physical activity and suicidal thoughts and behavior (Brosnahan et al., 2004; Brown and Blanton, 2002; Paffenbarger et al., 1994; Simon et al., 2004).

Physical Activity and Other Mental and Neurological Conditions

The literature addressing three additional conditions—schizophrenia, pain disorders, and self variables (e.g., self-concept, self-efficacy, self-esteem)—was not examined. The size of the literature is very small for schizophrenia and large for the other two conditions. Each of these conditions is an important topic that might merit further attention. In discussion, it was pointed out that the lifetime prevalence of low back pain is higher than 50 percent, that physical inactivity is a risk factor for low back pain (Vuori, 2001), and that a meta-analysis of 61 randomized controlled trials showed that exercise was more effective than usual care by the general practitioner and just as effective as conventional physical therapy for chronic low back pain (Hayden et al., 2005).

Concluding Remarks

Dr. O'Connor provided a qualitative summary of the size and quality of the evidence about the mental and neurological conditions he covered. For anxiety, depression, alcohol use, and smoking, the size of the literature is large and its quality is high to very high. A moderate amount of high-quality information is available about sleep, Alzheimer's disease, and feelings of fatigue. For the other conditions, the size of the literature is small and the quality is low to moderate.

PHYSICAL ACTIVITY AND DIABETES AND OTHER METABOLIC DISORDERS

Presenter: Judith G. Regensteiner[1]

Dr. Regensteiner stated that a wealth of strong data is available to support the use of physical activity in the prevention and treatment of type 2 diabetes mellitus. This presentation began with background information and then covered physiological studies, observational studies, randomized controlled trials, and meta-analyses related to physical activity and type 2 diabetes mellitus.

Background

Diabetes is a public health problem in the United States: approximately 21 million children and adults—7 percent of the population—have diabetes, but only about 14.6 million have been diagnosed (Sigal et al., 2006). A large majority of the people with diabetes have type 2 diabetes. The estimated number of persons with prediabetes is 54 million. The prevalence of diabetes is lower among Caucasians than among persons of some other racial/ethnic groups. Among persons with type 2 diabetes, two of three deaths are caused by CVD, myocardial infarction, or stroke. Figure 2-5 illustrates that men and women with diabetes have substantially higher mortality from heart disease than do persons without diabetes.

---

[1]Dr. Regensteiner acknowledged assistance from Richard Hammon, M.D., Dr.P.H. and Steven N. Blair, P.E.D.

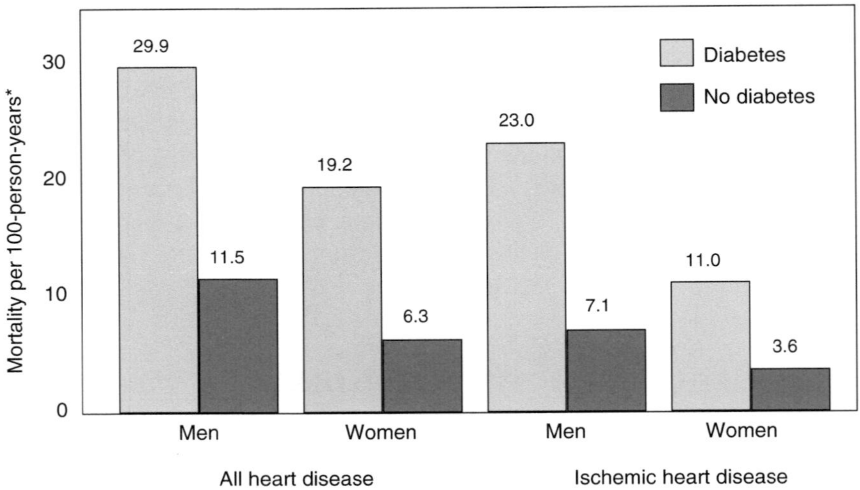

FIGURE 2-5 Mortality due to heart disease in men and women with or without diabetes.
NOTE: *Age-adjusted.
SOURCE: Adapted from Gu et al. (1998). Reprinted with permission from *The American Diabetes Association.* Copyright ©1998 American Diabetes Association. From *Diabetes Care*, Vol. 21, 1998; 1138–1145.

Compared with people without diabetes, people with diabetes have a higher prevalence of a number of conditions such as

- hypertension,
- blood lipid abnormalities (Sigal et al., 2006), and
- reduced exercise capacity (Regensteiner et al., 1998), including lower maximal oxygen consumption (VO_2max) and submaximal measures of cardiorespiratory fitness.

Impaired glucose metabolism, hyperinsulinemia, and increased insulin resistance are associated with sedentary behavior among those with diabetes and among those with prediabetes.

Physical activity can attenuate adverse effects in the progression from normal glucose metabolism to clinical type 2 diabetes and various complications, as shown in Figure 2-6. In contrast, physical inactivity accelerates these unfavorable metabolic and cardiovascular events.

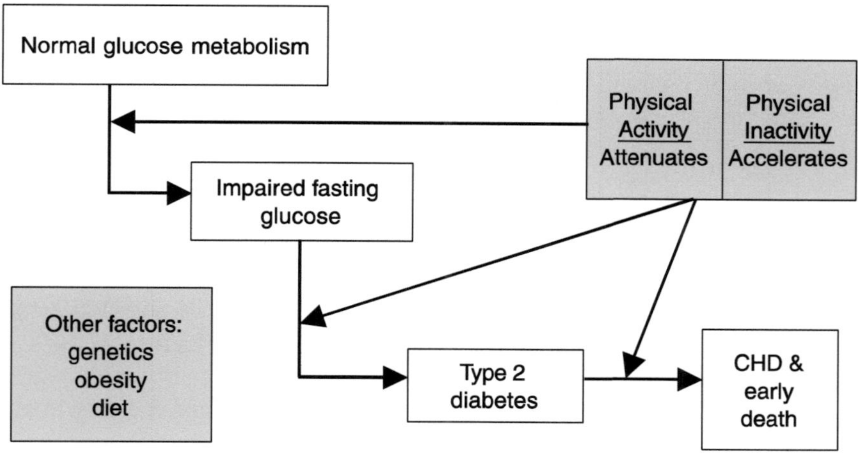

FIGURE 2-6 Relationship of physical activity with the progression from normal glucose metabolism to clinical type 2 diabetes and increased risk of cardiovascular diseases and other complications.
NOTE: CHD = coronary heart disease.
SOURCE: LaMonte et al. (2005a). Reprinted, with permission, from LaMonte MJ, Blair SN, and Church TS. Physical activity and diabetes prevention. *J Appl Physiol* 99:1205–1213, 2005.

Biological mechanisms by which physical activity may enhance metabolic and cardiovascular health and thereby confer protection against the negative effects of diabetes include structural and biochemical changes in skeletal muscle; improved maximal oxygen uptake and functional capacity, lipid factors, hepatic secretions, counterregulatory hormone concentrations or activity; and improvements in comorbid conditions (LaMonte et al. 2005a).

Physiological Data

A recent meta-analysis (Thomas et al., 2006) provides evidence that regular moderate intensity exercise benefits cardiorespiratory fitness in persons with diabetes and that higher intensity exercise would have an even greater effect. Even a single bout of moderate exercise has a profound effect on glucose metabolism that may last up to about 18 hours (Devlin et al., 1987). In addition, repeated bouts of exercise appear to have a cumulative beneficial effect on glucose metabolism. Exercise training in persons with diabetes also has a very significant effect in terms of improving VO_2max, measures of submaximal exercise performance, and other measures of fitness (Brandenburg et al., 1999).

Observational Studies of Diabetes Prevention

Large observational studies that assessed physical activity using questionnaires all suggest a benefit of increasing levels of physical activity for preventing diabetes (Helmrich et al., 1991; Hsia et al., 2005; Manson et al., 1991). Data from the British Regional Heart Study (Wannamethee et al., 2000), Iowa Women's Health Study (Folsom et al., 2000), and Study of Eastern Finns (Hu et al., 2003) provide additional supportive evidence. Similarly, observational studies that assessed physical activity with objective measures of cardiopulmonary fitness reported that better fitness reduced the risk of developing diabetes (Lynch et al., 1996; Wei et al., 1999).

Randomized Controlled Trials of Type 2 Diabetes Prevention

One of the earliest trials (Cederholm, 1985) demonstrated that diet plus exercise reduced the risk of developing diabetes. A trial in China (Pan et al., 1997) included an exercise treatment arm and found that even modest changes in exercise without change in diet reduced the risk of developing diabetes. The Diabetes Prevention Study in Finland (Eriksson et al., 1999; Tuomilehto et al., 2001) and the Diabetes Prevention Program in the United States (Knowler et al., 2002) provide strong evidence that intensive lifestyle modifications, including diet and exercise interventions, reduce the risk of developing diabetes. In the Diabetes Prevention Program study, weight loss was the dominant predictor of a reduced incidence of diabetes. However, both diet and physical activity predicted weight loss, and physical activity had a strong independent effect. Subsequently, studies in India (Ramachandran et al., 2006) and in Japan (Kosaka et al., 2005) provide similar results, including the independent effect of physical activity (Hamman et al., 2006).

Dose–Response Data

According to the Nurses Health Study (Hu et al., 1999), the Iowa Women's Health Study (Folsom et al., 2000), and the Study of Eastern Finns (Hu et al., 2003), approximately 30 minutes of moderate intensity exercise at least 5 days per week provides a substantial (25 percent to 36 percent) reduction in the risk of type 2 diabetes mellitus.

Studies of Cardiovascular Event Prevention Among Persons with Type 2 Diabetes

Among persons with diabetes, observational studies have shown that those who exercise or are more fit have a reduced risk of cardiovascular morbidity and mortality than do less active or less fit individuals (Blair et al., 1989; Gregg et al., 2003; Hu et al., 2001, 2004; Tanasescu et al., 2003). Data from the Diabetes Prevention Study in Finland show that all types of physical activity (e.g., recreational and occupational) are beneficial in reducing cardiovascular events and mortality (Hu et al., 2004).

Physical Activity and Other Metabolic Disorders

In a recent review, Bassuk and Manson (2005) report that body weight maintenance, insulin sensitivity and glycemic control, blood pressure, dyslipidemia, and inflammation and endothelial function all are impacted by the level of physical activity. In the Diabetes Prevention Program, the risk of developing the metabolic syndrome was lower for the lifestyle (diet and exercise) group than for the metformin (drug treatment) group or the placebo group (Orchard et al., 2005).

Very few studies have addressed physical activity and type 1 diabetes mellitus, a condition that is much less prevalent than type 2 diabetes. Cross-sectional studies report correlations between glycemic control and aerobic fitness or physical activity, and the few prospective trials provide equivocal data with regard to glycemic control (Riddell and Iscoe, 2006)—in part because of the danger of hypoglycemia.

Concluding Remarks

Dr. Regensteiner emphasized the strong evidence indicating that physical activity and moderate intensity exercise have a major role in the prevention of type 2 diabetes and in the prevention of CVD events and death among people with type 2 diabetes. In addition, physical activity and regular exercise are very important in the treatment of type 2 diabetes. Areas requiring additional study include both the causes and treatments of exercise impairments (that is, reduced ability to exercise) associated with type 1 and type 2 diabetes, and exercise and type 2 diabetes in children and adolescents.

DISCUSSION

Mechanisms of Action of Exercise in Diabetes

Discussant: Laurie J. Goodyear

An understanding of how exercise results in health benefits can be helpful in developing prescriptions for exercise. Dr. Goodyear provided an example relating to diabetes. Exercise works to promote the uptake of glucose by the muscle by a mechanism that is completely different from that of insulin. In particular, exercise appears to work through a protein called AMP-activated protein kinase (AMPK). Metformin, the leading diabetes drug, seems to work in the same way. A major question from people with diabetes and from medical students is, "How much exercise is needed to gain a physiological effect that promotes glucose uptake into the muscle and thereby reduce the need for medication?"

Physical Activity and Cognition

Discussant: Bradley Hatfield
(Presented by Rodney K. Dishman)

Physical activity and cognition is an emerging area of study that shows much promise. The measurement of mental function is challenging. Hendrie et al. (2006) defined elements of the cognitive domain, which range from intelligence to the executive functions of problem solving and planning. The National Institutes of Health's Cognitive and Emotional Health Project has the goal of identifying factors that can help people maintain or enhance their cognitive and emotional health as they grow older.

Evidence is accruing that physical activity is linked to cognitive ability and decline, but it is not yet sufficient for definitive conclusions. Not all areas of the brain age at the same rate, and executive processes are at special risk. In a summary of 18 randomized exercise intervention studies on cognitive function in persons age 55 and older, Colcombe and Kramer (2003) reported an overall effect size of 0.48, but the effect size varied for different functions. Thus, the type of task needs careful attention.

Genetic factors also need to be considered to account for variations in central nervous system adaptations to exercise. A preliminary study (Schuit et al., 2001) suggests that physical activity decreases the risk of cognitive decline among those with a specific genetic predisposition for cognitive decline. Measurement specificity is another issue. One may be unable to see effects at the behavioral level because of strategic compensation by the central nervous system. Neuroimaging and genetics studies may be helpful in identifying "invisible" brain ailments and their relationship to physical activity.

Group Discussion

Moderator: James R. Morrow

During the group discussion, points raised by participants included the following:

- Randomized controlled trials address effects of exercise on risk factors for CVD, such as blood pressure, and on mechanisms such as fibrinolytic activity and flow-mediated dilation.
- Evidence regarding the acute benefits of single bouts of exercise merits consideration. Single bouts of exercise elicit most of the benefits in terms of glucose homeostasis. Persons with diabetes may need to be conditioned to be able to complete an acute bout of exercise that is long enough to have an impact on glucose metabolism.

- Studies by Castaneda et al. (2002) and by Dunstan et al., (2002) address resistance training and type 2 diabetes, reduced blood pressure, improved muscle mass, reduced visceral fat, and improved glucose control.
- Consideration needs to be given to dose–response data. The dose includes the frequency and quantity of exercise, how it is integrated into one's lifestyle, and weekend or leisure-time exercise habits, among other factors. Dr. Andrea Dunn's randomized controlled trial related to depression used five different exercise doses. William Krause's work with the Studies of Targeted Risk Reduction Interventions through Defined Exercise may be useful.
- At least two prospective studies, including research from the Framingham Study by Chaisson et al. (1999), address the relationship between muscle weakness and the risk of developing osteoarthritis.
- A guidelines process could have many positive effects. The process needs to consider understandability, ease of use, relationships with the built environment, and the target audience. Guidelines could focus on health promotion and disease prevention, but probably there is sufficient evidence to focus on guidance for people with currently active disease as well. Moreover, there is literature on interventions to help people increase their physical activity. Emphasis was placed on presenting the information in a way that leads to the adoption and maintenance of physically active lifestyles.

REFERENCES

Abbott R, White LR, Ross GW, Masaki GH, Curb JD, Petrovitch H. 2004. Walking and dementia in physically capable elderly men. *J Am Med Assoc* 292(12):1447–1453.

Adlard PA, Perreau VM, Pop V, Cotman CW. 2005. Voluntary exercise decreases amyloid load in a transgenic model of Alzheimer's disease. *J Neurosci* 25(17):4217–4221.

Akerstedt T, Knutsson A, Westerholm P, Theorell T, Alfredsson L, Kecklund G. 2002. Sleep disturbances, work stress and work hours: A cross-sectional study. *J Psychosom Res* 53(3):741–748.

Andersen LB, Schnohr P, Schroll M, Hein HO. 2000. All-cause mortality associated with physical activity during leisure time, work, sports, and cycling to work. *Arch Intern Med* 160(11):1621–1628.

Arciero PJ, Vukovich MD, Holloszy JO, Racette SB, Kohrt WM. 1999. Comparison of short-term diet and exercise on insulin action in individuals with abnormal glucose tolerance. *J Appl Physiol* 86(6):1930–1935.

Barlow CE, LaMonte MJ, FitzGerald SJ, Kampert JB, Perrin JL, Blair SN. 2006. Cardiorespiratory fitness is an independent predictor of hypertension incidence among initially normotensive healthy women. *Am J Epidemiol* 163(2):142–150.

Bassuk SS, Manson JE. 2005. Epidemiological evidence for the role of physical activity in reducing risk of type 2 diabetes and cardiovascular disease. *J Appl Physiol* 99(3):1193–1204.

Baumert PW, Henderson JM, Thompson NJ. 1998. Health risk behaviors of adolescents participants in organized sports. *J Adolesc Health* 22(6):460–465.

Benington JH, Heller HC. 1995. Restoration of brain energy metabolism as the function of sleep. *Prog Neurobiol* 45(4):347–360.

Blair SN, Jacobs Jr DR, Powell KE. 1985. Relationships between exercise or physical activity and other health behaviors. *Public Health Rep* 100(2): 172–180.

Blair SN, Kohl HW III, Paffenbarger RS Jr, Clark DG, Cooper KH, Gibbons LW. 1989. Physical fitness and all-cause mortality. A prospective study of healthy men and women. *J Am Med Assoc* 262(17):2395–2401.

Blair SN, Kampert JB, Kohl HW III, Barlow CE, Macera CA, Paffenbarger RS Jr, Gibbons LW. 1996. Influences of cardiorespiratory fitness and other precursors on cardiovascular disease and all-cause mortality in men and women. *J Am Med Assoc* 276(3):205–210.

Blair SN, Wei M. 2000. Sedentary habits, health, and function in older women and men. *Am J Health Prom* 15(1):1–8.

Bonaiuti D, Shea B, Iovine R, Negrini S, Robinson V, Kemper HC, Wells G, Tugwell P, Cranney A. 2002. Exercise for preventing and treating osteoporosis in postmenopausal women. *Cochrane Database Syst Rev* CD000333. [Online]. Available: http://www.update-software.com/ABSTRACTS/AB000333.htm [accessed November 15, 2006].

Boyle RG, O'Connor P, Pronk N, Tan A. 2000. Health behaviors of smokers, ex-smokers and never smokers in an HMO. *Prev Med* 31(2):177–182.

Brandenburg SL, Bauer TA, Reusch JEB, Hiatt WR, Regensteiner JG. 1999. Effects of exercise training on oxygen uptake kinetic responses in women with type 2 diabetes mellitus. *Diabetes Care* 22(10):1640–1646.

Broe GA 1990. A case-control study of Alzheimer's disease in Australia. *Neurology* 40(11):1698–1707.

Broocks A, Bandelow B, Pekrun G, George A, Meyer T, Bartmann U, Hillmer-Vogel U, Rüther E. 1998. Comparison of aerobic exercise, clomipramine, and placebo in the treatment of panic disorder. *Am J Psychiatry* 155(5):603–609.

Brosnahan J, Steffen LM, Lytle L, Patterson J, Boostrom A. 2004. The relation between physical activity and mental health among Hispanic and non-Hispanic white adolescents. *Arch Pediatr Adolesc Med* 158(8):818–823.

Brown DR, Blanton CJ. 2002. Physical activity, sports participation, and suicidal behavior among college students. *Med Sci Sports Exerc* 34(7):1087–1096.

Castaneda C, Layne J, Munoz-Orians L, Gordon P, Walsmith J, Foldvari M, Roubenoff R, Tucker K, Nelson M. 2002. High-intensity progressive resistance exercise training in Hispanic older adults with type 2 diabetes: A randomized controlled trial. *Diabetes Care* 25(12):2335–2341.

Cederholm J. 1985. Findings in a health survey of middle-aged subjects in Uppsala 1981-82. Risk factors for diabetes mellitus and cardiovascular disease. *Ups J Med Sci* 90(3):201–227.

Chaisson CE, Zhang Y, Sharma L, Kannel W, Felson DT. 1999. Grip strength and the risk of developing radiographic hand osteoarthritis: Results from the Framingham Study. *Arthritis Rheum* 42(1):33–38.

Chambliss HO, Van Hoomissen JD, Holmes PV, Bunnell BN, Dishman RK. 2004. Effects of chronic activity wheel running and imipramine on masculine copulatory behavior after olfactory bulbectomy. *Physiol Behav* 82(4): 593–600.

Chen H, Zhang SM, Schwarzschild MA, Hernan MA, Ascherio A. 2005. Physical activity and the risk of Parkinson's disease. *Neurology* 64(4):664–669.

Cohen AD, Tillerson JL, Smith AD, Schallert T, Zigmond MJ 2003. Neuroprotective effects of prior limb use in 6-hydroxydopamine-treated rats: Possible role of GDNF. *J Neurochem* 85(2):299–305.

Colcombe S, Kramer AF. 2003. Fitness effects on the cognitive function of older adults: A meta-analytic study. *Psychol Sci* 14(2):125–130.

De Rijk MC, Rocca WA, Anderson DW, Melcon MO, Breteler MM, Maraganore DM. 1997. A population perspective on diagnostic criteria for Parkinson's disease. *J Neurol Neurosurg Psychiat* 62(1):10–15.

Devlin JT, Hirshman M, Horton ED, Horton ES. 1987. Enhanced peripheral and splanchnic insulin sensitivity in NIDDM men after single bout of exercise. *Diabetes* 36:434–439.

Dishman RK. 1997. Brain monoamines, exercise, and behavioral stress: Animal models. *Med Sci Sports Exerc* 29(1):63–74.

Dunn AL, Trivedi MH, O'Neal HA. 2001. Physical activity dose-response effects on outcomes of depression and anxiety. *Med Sci Sports Exerc* 33(6 Suppl):S587–S597.

Dunn AL, Trivedi MH, Kampert JB, Clark CG, Chambliss HO. 2005. Exercise treatment for depression: Efficacy and dose response. *Am J Prev Med* 28(1):1–8.

Dunstan DW, Daly RM, Owen N, Jolley D, De Courten M, Shaw J, Zimmet P. 2002. High-intensity resistance training improves glycemic control in older patients with type 2 diabetes. *Diabetes Care* 25(10):1729–1736.

Epstein L, Miller GJ, Stitt FW, Morris JN. 1976. Vigorous exercise in leisure time, coronary risk-factors, and resting electrocardiogram in middle-aged male civil servants. *Br Heart J* 38(4):403–409.

Erikssen G, Liestol K, Bjornholt J, Thaulow E, Sandvik L, Erikssen J. 1998. Changes in physical fitness and changes in mortality. *Lancet* 352(9130): 759–762.

Eriksson J, Lindstrom J, Valle T, Aunola S, Hamalainen H, Ilanne-Parikka P, Keinanen-Kiukaanniemi S, Laakso M, Lauhkonen M, Lehto P, Lehtonen A, Louheranta A, Mannelin M, Martikkala V, Rastas M, Sundvall J, Turpeinen A, Viljanen T, Uusitupa M, Tuomilehto J. 1999. Prevention of type II diabetes in subjects with impaired glucose tolerance: the Diabetes Prevention Study (DPS) in Finland. Study design and 1-year interim report on the feasibility of the lifestyle intervention programme. *Diabetologia* 42(7):793–801.

Farrell SW, Jurca R, Cortese GM, Blair SN, LaMonte MJ. 2006. The relation of cardiorespiratory fitness and adiposity with cancer mortality in men. *Med Sci Sports Exerc* 38(5):S425.

Feskanich D, Willett W, Colditz G. 2002. Walking and leisure-time activity and risk of hip fracture in postmenopausal women. *J Am Med Assoc* 288(18):2300–2306.

Fisher BM, Petzinger GM, Nixon K, Hogg E, Bremmer S, Meshul CK, Jakowec MW. 2004. Exercise-induced behavioral recovery and neuroplasticitiy in the 1-methyl-4-pheny-1,2,3,6-tetralhydropyridine-lesioned mouse basal ganglia. *J Neurosci Res* 77(3):378–390.

Folsom AR, Kushi LH, Hong CP. 2000. Physical activity and incident diabetes mellitus in postmenopausal women. *Am J Public Health* 90(1):134–138.

Friedland RP, Fritsch T, Smyth KA, Koss E, Lerner AJ, Chen CH, Petot GJ, Debanne SM. 2001. Patients with Alzheimer's disease have reduced activities in midlife compared with healthy control-group members. *Proc Natl Acad Sci* 98(6):3440–3445.

Frigerio R, Elbaz A, Sanft KR, Peterson BJ, Bower JH, Ahlskog JE, Grossardt BR, de Andrade M, Maraganore DM, Rocca WA. 2005. Education and occupations preceding Parkinson disease: A population-based case-control study. *Neurology* 65(10):1575–1583.

Fulcher KY, White PD. 1997. Randomised controlled trial of graded exercise in patients with the chronic fatigue syndrome. *BMJ* 314(7095):1647–1652.

Fulk LJ, Stock HS, Lynn A, Marshall J, Wilson MA, Hand GA. 2004. Chronic physical exercise reduces anxiety-like behavior in rats. *Int J Sports Med* 25(1):78–82.

Garg PK, Tian L, Criqui MH, Liu K, Ferrucci L, Guralnik JM, Tan J, McDermott MM. 2006. Physical activity during daily life and mortality in patients with peripheral arterial disease. *Circulation* 114(3):242–248.

Gregg EW, Gerzoff RB, Caspersen CJ, Williamson DF, Narayan KM. 2003. Relationship of walking to mortality among US adults with diabetes. *Arch Intern Med* 163(12):1440–1447.

Guilleminault C, Clerk A, Black J, Labanowski M, Pelayo R, Claman D. 1995. Nondrug treatment trials in psychophysiologic insomnia. *Arch Intern Med* 155(8):838–844.

Gu K, Cowie CC, Harris MI. 1998. Mortality in adults with and without diabetes in a national cohort of the U.S. population, 1971-1993. *Diabetes Care* 21(7):1138–1145.

Haddock CK, Klesges RC, Talcott GW, Lando H, Stein RJ. 1998. Smoking prevalence and risk factors for smoking in a population of United States Air Force basic trainees. *Tobacco Control* 7(3):232–235.

Hambrecht R, Walther C, Mobius-Winkler S, Gielen S, Linke A, Conradi K, Erbs S, Kluge R, Kendziorra K, Sabri O, Sick P, Schuler G. 2004. Percutaneous coronary angioplasty compared with exercise training in patients with stable coronary artery disease: A randomized trial. *Circulation* 109(11):1371–1378.

Hamman R, Wing R, Edelstein S, Lachin J, Bray G, Delahanty L, Hoskin M, Kriska A, Mayer Davis E, Pi-Sunyer X, Regensteiner JG, Venditti B. 2006. Effect of weight loss with lifestyle intervention on risk of diabetes in the Diabetes Prevention Program (DPP). *Diabetes Care* 29(9):2102–2107.

Hawkins SA, Marcell TJ, Victoria JS, Wiswell RA. 2001. A longitudinal assessment of change in VO2max and maximal heart rate in master athletes. *Med Sci Sports Exerc* 33(10):1744–1750.

Hayden JA, van Tulder MW, Malmivaara AV, Koes BW. 2005. Meta-analysis: Exercise therapy for nonspecific low back pain. *Ann Intern Med* 142(9): 765–775.

Helmrich SP, Ragland DR, Leung RW, Paffenbarger RS Jr. 1991. Physical activity and reduced occurrence of non-insulin-dependent diabetes mellitus. *N Engl J Med* 325(3):147–152.

Hendrie HC, Albert MS, Butters MA, Gao S, Knopman DS, Launer LJ, Yaffe K, Cuthbert BN, Edwards E, Wagster MV. 2006. The NIH Cognitive and Emotional Health Project: Report of the Critical Evaluation Study Committee. *Alzheimer's Dementia* 2:12–32.

Herbert LE, Beckett LA, Scherr PA, Evans DA. 2001. Annual incidence of Alzheimer disease in the United States projected to the years 2000 through 2050. *Alzheimer Dis Assoc Disord* 15(4):169–173.

Heyn P, Abreu BC, Ottenbacher KJ. 2004. The effects of exercise training on elderly persons with cognitive impairment and dementia: A meta-analysis. *Arch Phys Med Rehabil* 85(10):1694–1704.

Hickey N, Mulcahy R, Bourke GJ, Graham I, Wilson-Davis K. 1975. Study of coronary risk factors related to physical activity in 15 171 men. *Br Med J* 3(5982):507–509.

Holloszy JO, Kohrt WM. 1995. Exercise. In: Masoro EJ, ed. *Handbook of Physiology—Aging*. New York: Oxford University Press. Pp. 633–666.

Holme I, Helgeland A, Hjermann I, Leren P, Lund-Larsen PG. 1981. Physical activity at work and at leisure in relation to coronary risk factors and social class. A 4-year mortality follow-up. The Oslo study. *Acta Med Scand* 209(4):277–283.

Holmes MD, Chen WY, Feskanich D, Kroenke CH, Colditz GA. 2005. Physical activity and survival after breast cancer diagnosis. *J Am Med Assoc* 293(20):2479–2486.

Hsia J, Wu L, Allen C, Oberman A, Lawson WE, Torrens J, Safford M, Limacher MC, Howard BV. 2005. Physical activity and diabetes risk in postmenopausal women. *Am J Prev Med* 28(1):19–25.

Hu FB, Sigal RJ, Rich-Edwards JW, Colditz GA, Solomon CG, Willett WC, Speizer FE, and Manson JE. 1999. Walking compared with vigorous physical activity and risk of type 2 diabetes in women: A prospective study. *J Am Med Assoc* 282(15):1433–1439.

Hu FB, Stampfer MJ, Solomon C, Liu S, Colditz GA, Speizer FE, Willett WC, Manson JE. 2001. Physical activity and risk for cardiovascular events in diabetic women. *Ann Intern Med* 134(2):96–105.

Hu G, Qiao Q, Silventoinen K, Eriksson JG, Jousilahti P, Lindstrom J, Valle TT, Nissinen A, Tuomilehto J. 2003. Occupational, commuting, and leisure-time physical activity in relation to risk for type 2 diabetes in middle-aged Finnish men and women. *Diabetologia* 46:322–329.

Hu G, Eriksson J, Barengo NC, Lakka TA, Valle TT, Nissinen A, Jousilahti P, Tuomilehto J. 2004. Occupational, commuting, and leisure-time physical activity in relation to total and cardiovascular mortality among Finnish subjects with type 2 diabetes. *Circulation* 110(6):666–673.

Jason LA, Richman JA, Rademaker AW, Jordan KM, Plioplys AV, Taylor RR, McCready W, Huang CF, Plioplys S. 1999. A community-based study of chronic fatigue syndrome. *Arch Intern Med* 159(18):2129–2137.

Jones G, Bennell K, Cicuttini FM. 2003. Effect of physical activity on cartilage development in healthy kids. *Br J Sports Med* 37(5):382–383.

Katzmarzyk PT, Church TS, Blair SN. 2004. Cardiorespiratory fitness attenuates the effects of the metabolic syndrome on all-cause and cardiovascular disease mortality in men. *Arch Intern Med* 164(10):1092–1097.

Kawamoto R, Yoshida O, Oka Y, Takagi Y. 2004. Risk factors for insomnia in community-dwelling older persons. *Geriat Gerontol Internat* 4(3):163–168.

Kessler RC, Coccaro EF, Fava M, Jaeger S, Jin R, Walters 2006. The prevalence and correlates of DSM-IV intermittent explosive disorder in the National Comorbidity Survey Replication. *Arch Gen Psychiatry* 63(6):669–678.

Kim K, Uchiyama M, Okawa M, Liu X, Ogihara R. 2000. An epidemiological study of insomnia among the Japanese general population. *Sleep* 23(1):1–7.

King AC, Oman RF, Brassington GS, Bliwise DL, Haskell WL. 1997. Moderate-intensity exercise and self-rated quality of sleep in older adults. A randomized controlled trial. *J Am Med Assoc* 277(1):32–37.

King AC, Baumann K, O'Sullivan P, Wilcox S, Castro C. 2002. Effects of moderate-intensity exercise on physiological, behavioral, and emotional responses to family caregiving: A randomized controlled trial. *J Gerontology A Biol Sci Med Sci* 57(1):M26–M36.

Knowler WC, Barrett-Connor E, Fowler SE, Hamman RF, Lachin JM, Walker EA, Nathan DM, Diabetes Prevention Program Research Group. 2002. Reduction in the incidence of type 2 diabetes with lifestyle intervention or metformin. *N Engl J Med* 346(6):393–403.

Kondo K, Niino M, Shido K. 1994. A case-control study of Alzheimer's disease in Japan—significance of lifestyles. *Dementia* 5(6):314–326.

Kosaka K, Noda M, Kuzuya T. 2005. Prevention of type 2 diabetes by lifestyle intervention: A Japanese trial in IGT males. *Diabetes Res Clin Pract* 67(2):152–162.

Kravitz HM, Ganz PA, Bromberger J, Powell LH, Sutton-Tyrrell K, Meyer PM. 2003. Sleep difficulty in women at midlife: A community survey of sleep and the menopausal transition. *Menopause* 10(1):19–28.

Kuopio AM, Marttila RJ, Helenius H, Rinne UK. 1999. Environmental risk factors in Parkinson's disease. *Movement Disord* 14(6):928–939.

Kyle UG, Genton L, Gremion G, Slosman DO, Pichard C. 2004. Aging, physical activity and height-normalized body composition parameters. *Clin Nutr* 23(1):79–88.

LaMonte MJ, Blair SN, Church TS. 2005a. Physical activity and diabetes prevention. *J Appl Physiol* 99(3):1205–1213.

LaMonte MJ, Jurca R, Kampert JB, Gibbons LW, Church TS, FitzGerald SJ, Barlow CE, Nichaman MZ, Blair SN, Radford NB. 2005b. Exercise tolerance adds prognostic value to the Framingham Risk Score in asymptomatic women and men. *Circulation* 112(17):SII–829.

LaMonte MJ, FitzGerald SJ, Church TS, Barlow CE, Radford NB, Levine BD, Pippin JJ, Gibbons LW, Blair SN, Nichaman MZ. 2005c. Coronary artery calcium score and coronary heart disease events in a large cohort of asymptomatic men and women. *Am J Epidemiol*162(5):421–429.

LaMonte MJ, FitzGerald SJ, Levine BD, Church TS, Kampert JB, Nichaman MZ, Gibbons LW, Blair SN. 2006. Coronary artery calcium, exercise tolerance, and CHD events in asymptomatic men. *Atherosclerosis* 189(1):157–162.

Larson EB, Wang L, Bowen JD, McCormick WC, Teri L, Crane P, Kukull W. 2006. Exercise is associated with reduced risk for incident dementia among persons 65 years of age and older. *Ann Intern Med* 144(2):73–81.

Law MR, Wald NJ, Meade TW. 1991. Strategies for prevention of osteoporosis and hip fracture. *BMJ* 303(6800):453–459.

Lawlor DA, Hopker SW. 2001. The effectiveness of exercise as an intervention in the management of depression: Systematic review and meta-regression analysis of randomised controlled trials. *BMJ* 322(7289):763–767.

Lee CD, Blair, SN, Jackson, AS. 1999. Cardiorespiratory fitness, body composition, and all-cause and cardiovascular disease mortality in men. *Am J Clin Nutr* 69(3):373–380.

Lindsay J, Laurin D, Verreault R, Hebert R, Helliwell B, Hill GB, McDowell I. 2002. Risk factors for Alzheimer's disease: A prospective analysis from the Canadian Study of Health and Aging. *Am J Epidemiol* 156(5):445–452.

Littman A, Vitiello MV, Foster-Schubert K, Ulrich CM, Tworoger SS, Potter JD, Weigle DS, McTiernan A. 2006. Sleep, ghrelin, leptin and changes in body weight during a 1-year moderate-intensity physical activity intervention. *Int J Obesity* Aug 15. [Online]. Available: http://www.nature.com/ijo/journal/v30/n8/index.html. [accessed December 21, 2006].

Liu X, Uchiyama M, Okawa M, Kurita H. 2000. Prevalence and correlates of self-reported sleep problems among Chinese adolescents. *Sleep* 23(1):27–34.

Logroscino G, Sesso HD, Paffenbarger RS Jr, Lee IM. 2006. Physical activity and risk of Parkinson's disease: A prospective cohort study. *J Neurol Neurosury Psychiatry*. 77(12):1318–1322.

Lynch J, Helmrich SP, Lakka TA, Kaplan GA, Cohen RD, Salonen R, and Salonen JT. 1996. Moderately intense physical activities and high levels of cardiorespiratory fitness reduce the risk of non-insulin-dependent diabetes mellitus in middle-aged men. *Arch Intern Med* 156(12):1307–1314.

Manini TM, Everhart JE, Patel KV, Schoeller DA, Colbert LH, Visser M, Tylavsky F, Bauer DC, Goodpaster BH, Harris TB. 2006. Daily activity energy expenditure and mortality among older adults. *J Am Med Assoc* 296(2):171–179.

Manson JE, Rimm EB, Stampfer MJ, Colditz GA, Willett WC, Krolewski AS, Rosner B, Hennekens CH, and Speizer FE. 1991. Physical activity and incidence of non-insulin-dependent diabetes mellitus in women. *Lancet* 338(8770):774–778.

Manson JE, Nathan DM, Krolewski AS, Stampfer MJ, Willett WC, and Hennekens CH. 1992. A prospective study of exercise and incidence of diabetes among U.S. male physicians. *J Am Med Assoc* 268(1):63–67.

Manson JE, Greenland P, LaCroix AZ, Stefanick ML, Mouton CP, Oberman A, Perri MG, Sheps DS, Pettinger MB, Siscovick DS. 2002. Walking compared with vigorous exercise for the prevention of cardiovascular events in women. *N Engl J Med* 347(10):716–725.

Miyai I, Fujimoto Y, Yamamoto H, Ueda Y, Saito T, Nozaki S, Kang J. 2002. Long-term effect of body weight-supported treadmill training in Parkinson's disease: A randomized controlled trial. *Arch Phys Med Rehabil* 83(10):1370–1373.

Morgan K. 2003. Daytime activity and risk factors for late-life insomnia. *J Sleep Res* 12(3):231–238.

Morin CM, LeBlanc M, Daley M, Gregoire JP, Merette C. 2006. Epidemiology of insomnia: Prevalence, self-help treatments, consultations, and determinants of help-seeking behaviors. *Sleep Med* 7(2):123–130.

Morris JN, Heady JA, Raffle PA, Roberts CG, Parks JW. 1953. Coronary heart-disease and physical activity of work. *Lancet* 265(6795,6796):1053–1057, 1111–1120.

Moss-Morris R, Sharon C, Tobin R, Baldi JC. 2005. A randomized controlled graded exercise trial for chronic fatigue syndrome: Outcomes and mechanisms of change. *J Health Psychol* 10(2):245–259.

Mostert S, Kesslering J. 2002. Effects of a short-term exercise training program on aerobic fitness, fatigue, health perception and activity level of subjects with multiple sclerosis. *Multiple Sclerosis* 8(2):161–168.

Mukamal KJ, Ding EL, Djousse L. 2006. Alcohol consumption, physical activity, and chronic disease risk factors: A population-based cross-sectional survey. *BMC Public Health* 6:118.

Nasermoaddeli A, Sekine M, Kumari M, Chandola T, Marmot M, Kagamimori S. 2005. Association of sleep quality and free time leisure activities in Japanese and British civil servants. *J Occup Health* 47(5):384–390.

Newman AB, Simonsick EM, Naydeck BL, Boudreau RM, Kritchevsky SB, Nevitt MC, Pahor M, Satterfield S, Brach JS, Studenski SA, Harris TB. 2006. Association of long-distance corridor walk performance with mortality, cardiovascular disease, mobility limitation, and disability. *J Am Med Assoc* 295(17):2018–2026.

Ohayon MM. 2004. Interactions between sleep normative data and sociocultural characteristics in the elderly. *J Psychosom Res* 56(5):479–486.

Ohida T, Kamal AM, Uchiyama M, Kim K, Takemura S, Sone T, Ishii T. 2001. The influence of lifestyle and health status factors on sleep loss among the Japanese general population. *Sleep* 24(3):333–338.

Oken BS, Kishiyama S, Zajdel D, Bourdette D, Carlsen J, Haas M, Hugos C, Kraemer DF, Lawrence J, Mass M. 2004. Randomized controlled trial of yoga and exercise in multiple sclerosis. *Neurology* 62(11):2058–2064.

Oler MJ, Mainous AG III, Martin CA, Richardson E, Haney A, Wilson D, Adams T. 1994. Depression, suicidal ideation, and substance use among adolescents. Are athletes at less risk? *Arch Fam Med* 3(9):781–785.

Orchard TJ, Temprosa M, Goldberg R, Haffner S, Ratner R, Marcovina S, Fowler S, Diabetes Prevention Program Research Group. 2005. The effect of metformin and intensive lifestyle intervention on the metabolic syndrome: The Diabetes Prevention Program randomized trial. *Ann Intern Med* 19(142):611–619.

Paffenbarger RS, Hale WE. 1975. Work activity and coronary heart mortality. *N Engl J Med* 292(11):545–550.

Paffenbarger RS Jr, Lee IM, Leung R. 1994. Physical activity and personal characteristics associated with depression and suicide in American college men. *Acta Psychiatr Scand Suppl* 377:16–22.

Page RM, Hammermeister J, Scanlon A, Gilbert L. 1998. Is school sports participation a protective factor against adolescent health risk behaviors? *J Health Educ* 29:186–192.

Pan XR, Li GW, Hu YH, Wang JX, Yang WY, An ZX, Hu ZX, Lin J, Xiao JZ, Cao HB, Liu PA, Jiang XG, Jiang YY, Wang JP, Zheng H, Zhang H, Bennett PH, Howard BV. 1997. Effects of diet and exercise in preventing NIDDM in people with impaired glucose tolerance. The Da Qing IGT and Diabetes Study. *Diabetes Care* 20(4):537–544.

Pate RR, Heath GW, Dowda M, Trost SG. 1996. Associations between physical activity and other health behaviors in a representative sample of US adolescents. *Am J Public Health* 86(11):1577–1581.

Peppard PE, Young T. 2004. Exercise and sleep-disordered breathing: An association independent of body habitus. *Sleep* 27(3):480–484.

Petajan JH, Gappmaier E, White AT, Spencer MK, Mino L, Hicks RW. 1996. Impact of aerobic training on fitness and quality of life in multiple sclerosis. *Ann Neurol* 39(4):432–441.

Phillips B, Young T, Finn L, Asher K, Hening WA, Purvis C. 2000. Epidemiology of restless legs symptoms in adults. *Arch Intern Med* 160(14):2137–2141.

Podewils LJ, Guallar E, Kuller LH, Fried LP, Lopez OL, Carlson M, Lyketsos CG. 2005. Physical activity, APOE genotype, and dementia risk: Findings from the Cardiovascular Health Cognition Study. *Am J Epidemiol* 161(7):639–651.

Poulton NP, Muir G. 2005. Treadmill training ameliorates dopamine loss but not behavioral deficits in hemi-Parkinsonian rats. *Exp Neurol* 193(1):181–197.

Powell P, Bentall RP, Nye FJ, Edwards RH. 2001. Randomised controlled trial of patient education to encourage graded exercise in chronic fatigue syndrome. *BMJ* 322(7283):387–390.

Puetz TW, O'Connor PJ, Dishman RK. 2006. Effects of chronic exercise on feelings of energy and fatigue: A quantitative synthesis. *Psych Bull* 132(6):866–876.

Ramachandran A, Snehalatha C, Mary S, Mukesh B, Bhaskar AD, Vijay V; Indian Diabetes Prevention Programme (IDPP). 2006. The Indian Diabetes Prevention Programme shows that lifestyle modification and metformin prevent type 2 diabetes in Asian Indian subjects with impaired glucose tolerance (IDPP-1). *Diabetologia* 49(2):289–297.

Regensteiner JG, Bauer TA, Reusch JEB, Brandenburg SL, Sippel JT, Vogelsong AM, Smith S, Wolfel EE, Eckel RH, Hiatt WR. 1998. Abnormal oxygen uptake kinetic responses in women with type II diabetes mellitus. *J Appl Physiol* 85(1):310–317.

Reynolds P, Hurley SE, Hoggatt K, Anton-Culver H, Bernstein L, Deapen D, Peel D. 2004. Correlates of active and passive smoking in the California Teachers Study cohort. *J Women's Health* 13(7):778–790.

Riddell MC, Iscoe KE. 2006. Physical activity, sport, and pediatric diabetes. *Pediatr Diabetes* 7(1):60–70.

Roddy E, Zhang W, Doherty M, Arden NK, Barlow J, Birrell F, Carr A, Chakravarty K, Dickson J, Hay E, Hosie G, Hurley M, Jordan KM, McCarthy C, McMurdo M, Mockett S, O'Reilly S, Peat G, Pendleton A, Richards S. 2005. Evidence-based recommendations for the role of exercise in the management of osteoarthritis of the hip or knee--the MOVE consensus. *Rheumatology* 44(1):67–73.

Romberg A, Virtanen A, Ruutiainen J, Aunola S, Karppi SL, Vaara M, Surakka J, Pohjolainen T, Seppanen A. 2004. Effects of a 6-month exercise program on patients with multiple sclerosis. *Neurology* 63(11):2034–2038.

Romberg A, Virtanen A, Ruutiainen J. 2005. Long-term exercise improves functional impairment but not quality of life in multiple sclerosis. *J Neurology* 252(7):839–845.

Rovio S, Kareholt I, Helkala EL, Viitanen M, Winblad B, Tuomilehto J, Soininen H, Nissinen A, Kivipelto M. 2005. Leisure-time physical activity at midlife and the risk of dementia and Alzheimer's disease. *Lancet Neurol* 4(11):705–711.

Russo-Neustadt AA, Beard RC, Huang YM, Cotman CW. 2000. Physical activity and antidepressant treatment potentiate the expression of specific brain-derived neurotrophic factor transcripts in the rat hippocampus. *Neuroscience* 101(2):305–312.

Sasco AJ, Paffenbarger RS Jr, Gendre I, Wing AL. 1992. The role of physical exercise in the occurrence of Parkinson's disease. *Arch Neurol* 49(4):360–365.

Sawada SS, Muto T, Tanaka H, Lee IM, Paffenbarger RS Jr, Shindo M, Blair SN. 2003. Cardiorespiratory fitness and gastric cancer mortality: A prospective study of Japanese men. *Med Sci Sports Exerc* 34 (5 suppl):S25.

Scarmea N, Levy G, Tang MX, Manly J, Stern Y. 2001. Influence of leisure activity on the incidence of Alzheimer's disease. *Neurology* 57(12):2236–2242.

Schenkman M, Cutson TM, Kuchibhatla M, Chandler J, Pieper CF, Ray L, Laub KC. 1998. Exercise to improve spinal flexibility and function for people with Parkinson's disease: A randomized, controlled trial. *J Am Geriatr Soc* 46(10):1207–1216.

Schmitz-Hubsch T, Pyfer D, Kielwein K, Fimmers R, Klockgether T, Wullner U. 2006. Qigong exercise for the symptoms of Parkinson's disease: A randomized, controlled pilot study. *Mov Disord* 21(4):543–548.

Schuit AJ, Feskens EJ, Launer LJ, Kromhout D. 2001. Physical activity and cognitive decline, the role of the apolipoprotein e4 allele. *Med Sci Sports Exerc* 33(5):772–777.

Sherrill D, Sherrill DL, Kotchou K, Quan SF. 1998. Association of physical activity and human sleep disorders. *Arch Intern Med* 158(17):1894–1898.

Sigal RJ, Kenny GP, Wasserman DH, Castaneda-Sceppa C, White RD. 2006. Physical activity/exercise and type 2 diabetes: A consensus statement from the American Diabetes Association. *Diabetes Care* 29(6):1433–1438.

Simon TR, Powell KE, Swann AC. 2004. Involvement in physical activity and risk for nearly lethal suicide attempts. *Am J Prev Med* 27(4):310–315.

Simones EJ, Byers T, Coates RJ, Serdula MK, Mokdad AH, Heath GW. 1995. The association between leisure-time physical activity and dietary fat in American adults. *Am J Public Health* 85(2):240–244.

Singh N, Clements KM, Fiatarone MA. 1997. A randomized trial of the effect of exercise on sleep. *Sleep* 20(2):95–101.

Singh N, Stavrinos TM, Scarbek Y, Galambos G, Liber C, Fiatarone Singh MA. 2005. A randomized controlled trial of high versus low intensity weight training versus general practitioner care for clinical depression in older adults. *J Gerontol* 60(6):768–776.

Slaughter JR, Slaughter KA, Nichols D, Holmes SE, Martens MP. 2001. Prevalence, clinical manifestations, etiology, and treatment of depression in Parkinson's disease. *J Neuropsychiatry Clin Neurosci* 13(2):187–196.

Solari A, Filippini G, Gasco P, Colla L, Salmaggi A, La Mantia L, Farinotti M, Eoli M, Mendozzi L. 1999. Physical rehabilitation has a positive effect on disability in multiple sclerosis patients. *Neurology* 52(1):57–62.

Steptoe A, Wardle J, Fuller R, Holte A, Justo J, Sanderman R, Wichstrom L. 1997. Leisure-time physical exercise: Prevalence, attitudinal correlates, and behavioral correlates among young Europeans from 21 countries. *Prev Med* 26(6):845–854.

Stuifbergen AK, Blozis SA, Harrison TC, Becker HA. 2006. Exercise, functional limitations, and quality of life: A longitudinal study of persons with multiple sclerosis. *Arch Phys Med* 87(7):935–943.

Surkan PJ, Ryan LM, Bidwell HW, Brooks DR, Peterson KE, Gillman MW. 2005. Psychosocial correlates of leisure-time physical activity in urban working-class adults. *J Phys Activ Health* 2(4):395–409.

Tanasescu M, Leitzmann MF, Rimm EB, Hu FB. 2003. Physical activity in relation to cardiovascular disease and total mortality among men with type 2 diabetes. *Circulation* 107(19): 2435–2439.

Tillerson JL, Caudle WM, Reveron ME, Miller GW. 2003. Exercise induces behavioral recovery and attenuates neurochemical deficits in rodent models of Parkinson's disease. *Neuroscience* 119(3):899–911.

Thomas DE, Elliott EJ, Naughton GA. 2006. Exercise for type 2 diabetes mellitus (Cochrane Review). *Cochrane Database of Systematic Reviews* 3:CD002968.

Tomori M, Zalar B. 2000. Sport and physical activity as possible protective factors in relation to adolescent suicide attempts. *Inter J Sport Psychol* 31(3):405–413.

Tretli S, Bjartveit K, Foss OP, Haider T, Lund-Larsen PG. 1985. Intervention on cardiovascular disease risk factors in Finnmark county: Changes after a period of three years. The Cardiovascular Disease Study in Finnmark Couty, Norway. *Scand J Soc Med* 13(1):1–13.

Tsai CH, Lo SK, See LC, Chen HZ, Chen RS, Weng YH, Chang FC, Lu CS. 2002. Environmental risk factors of young onset Parkinson's disease: A case-control study. *Clin Neurol Neurosur* 104(4):328–333.

Tuomilehto J, Lindstrom J, Eriksson JG, Valle TT, Hamalainen H, Ilanne-Parikka P, Keinanen-Kiukaanniemi S, Laakso M, Louheranta A, Rastas M, Salminen V, Uusitupa M. 2001. Prevention of type 2 diabetes mellitus by changes in lifestyle among subjects with impaired glucose tolerance. *N Engl J Med* 344(18):1343–1350.

Turner CH, Robling AG. 2003. Designing exercise regimens to increase bone strength. *Exerc Sport Sci Rev* 31(1):45–50.

Tworoger S, Yasui Y, Vitiello MV, Schwartz RS, Ulrich CM, Aiello EJ, Irwin ML, Bowen D, Potter JD, McTiernan A. 2003. Effects of a year-long moderate-intensity exercise and a stretching intervention on sleep quality in postmenopausal women. *Sleep* 26(7):830–836.

Tynjala J, Kannas L, Levalahti E, Valimaa R. 1999. Perceived sleep quality and its precursors in adolescents. *Health Promot Internat* 14(2):155–166.

Unger JB. 1997. Physical activity, participation in team sports, and risk of suicidal behavior in adolescents. *Am J Health Promot* 12(2):90–93.

Ussher M. 2005. Exercise interventions for smoking cessation. *Cochrane Database Syst Rev* 25;(1):CD002295

van den Berg M, Dawes H, Wade DT, Newman M, Burridge J, Izadi H, Sackley CH. 2006. Treadmill training for individuals with multiple sclerosis: A pilot randomised trial. *J Neurol Neurosurg Psychiatry* 77(4):531–533.

van der Poest CE, van der Wiel H, Patka P, Roos JC, Lips P. 1999. Long-term consequences of fracture of the lower leg: Cross-sectional study and long-term longitudinal follow-up of bone mineral density in the hip after fracture of lower leg. *Bone* 24(2):131–134.

Van Hoomissen JD, Chambliss HO, Holmes PV, Dishman RK. 2003. Effects of chronic exercise and imipramine on mRNA for BDNF after olfactory bulbectomy in rat. *Brain Res* 974(1–2):228–235.

Van Reeth O, Sturis J, Byrne MM, Blackman JD, L'Hermite-Baleriaux M, Leproult R, Oliner C, Refetoff S, Turek FW, Van Cauter E. 1994. Nocturnal exercise phase delays circadian rhythms of melatonin and thyrotropin secretion in normal men. *Am J Physiol* 266(6 Pt 1):E964–E974.

Verghese J, Lipton RB, Katz MJ, Hall CB, Derby CA, Kuslansky G, Ambrose AF, Sliwinski M, Buschke H. 2003. Leisure activities and the risk of dementia in the elderly. *N Engl J Med* 348(25):2508–2516.

Vuori IM. 2001. Dose-response of physical activity and low back pain, osteoarthritis, and osteoporosis. *Med Sci Sports Exerc* 33(6 Suppl):S551–S586.

Wagner A, Simon C, Evans A, Ducimetiere P, Bongard V, Montaye M, Arveiler D, PRIME Study Group. 2003. Physical activity pattern in 50–59 year men in France and Northern Ireland. Associations with socio-economic status and health behavior. *Eur J Epidemiol* 18(4):321–329.

Wallace BA, Cumming RG. 2000. Systematic review of randomized trials of the effect of exercise on bone mass in pre- and postmenopausal women. *Calcif Tissue Int* 67(1):10–18.

Wallman KE, Morton AR, Goodman C, Grove R, Guilfoyle AM. 2004. Randomised controlled trial of graded exercise in chronic fatigue syndrome. *Med J Aust* 180(9):444–448.

Wannamethee SG, Shaper AG, Alberti KG. 2000. Physical activity, metabolic factors, and the incidence of coronary heart disease and type 2 diabetes. *Arch Intern Med* 160(14):2108–2116.

Ward KD, Vander Weg MW, Klesges RC, Kovach KW, Elrod MC, DeBon M, Haddock CK, Talcott GW, Lando HA. 2003. Characteristics of highly physically active smokers in a population of young adult military recruits. *Addict Behav* 28(8):1405–1418.

Wei M, Gibbons LW, Mitchell TL, Kampert JB, Lee CD, Blair SN. 1999. The association between cardiorespiratory fitness and impaired fasting glucose and type 2 diabetes mellitus in men. *Ann Intern Med* 130(2):89–96.

Wearden AJ, Morriss RK, Mullis R, Strickland PL, Pearson DJ, Appleby L, Campbell IT, Morris JA. 1998. Randomised, double-blind, placebo-controlled treatment trial of fluoxetine and graded exercise for chronic fatigue syndrome. *Br J Psychiatry* 172(6):485–490.

Westerterp KR. 2000. Daily physical activity, aging and body composition. *J Nutr Health Aging* 4(4):239–242.

Whang W, Manson JE, Hu FB, Chae CU, Rexrode KM, Willett WC, Stampfer MJ, Albert CM. 2006. Physical exertion, exercise, and sudden cardiac death in women. *J Am Med Assoc* 295(12):1399–1403.

Wiles CM, Newcombe RG, Fuller KJ, Shaw S, Furnival-Doran J, Pickersgill TP, Morgan A. 2001. Controlled randomised crossover trial of the effects of physiotherapy on mobility in chronic multiple sclerosis. *J Neurol Neurosurg Psychiatry* 70(2):174–179.

Wilson RS, Mendes De Leon CF, Barnes LL, Schneider JA, Bienias JL, Evans DA, Bennett DA. 2002a. Participation in cognitively stimulating activities and risk of incident Alzheimer disease. *J Am Med Assoc* 287(6):742–748.

Wilson RS, Bennett DA, Bienias JL, Aggarwal NT, Mendes De Leon CF, Morris MC, Schneider JA, Evans DA. 2002b. Cognitive activity and incident AD in a population-based sample of older persons. *Neurology* 59(12):1910–1914.

Wolf SA, Kronenberg G, Lehmann K, Blankenship A, Overall R, Staufenbiel M, Kempermann G. 2006. Cognitive and physical activity differently modulate disease progression in the amyloid precursor protein (APP)-23 model of Alzheimer's disease. *Biol Psychiatry* 60(12):1314–1323.

Yoshitake T, Kiyohara Y, Kato I, Ohmura T, Iwamoto H, Nakayama K, Ohmori S, Nomiyama K, Kawano H, Ueda K. 1995. Incidence and risk factors of vascular dementia and Alzheimer's disease in a defined elderly Japanese population: The Hisayma Study. *Am Acad Neurol* 45(6):1161–1168.

Youngstedt SD. 2005. Effects of exercise on sleep. *Clin Sports Med* 24(2): 355–365.

3

Physical Activity, Obesity, and Weight Management

The effects of physical activity have been investigated in relation to weight loss, weight loss maintenance, and the prevention of weight gain. This workshop session included a presentation on those topics followed by a discussion period. This chapter includes a review of the evidence on effects of physical activity in weight management; a brief discussion of aging, inactivity, and obesity; additional information from epidemiological studies; and a brief summary of major points raised during the group discussion.

EFFECTS OF PHYSICAL ACTIVITY ON WEIGHT LOSS, WEIGHT LOSS MAINTENANCE, AND THE PREVENTION OF WEIGHT GAIN

Presenter: Joseph E. Donnelly

This presentation provided background information on physical activity and weight management, and also addressed various types of evidence related to physical activity for weight loss and for the prevention of weight gain.

Background

The general concept of physical activity and weight management is straightforward:

- Physical activity expends energy
- Energy expenditure can produce a negative energy balance
- Weight loss occurs during a negative energy balance

Many compensatory mechanisms can occur, however, when one increases physical activity. These include changes in diet, spontaneous activity, resting metabolism, and others. Thus an important question is how to create an energy gap that is effective for weight management (including weight maintenance or weight loss).

Evidence that Physical Activity Will Alter Energy Balance and Provide Weight Loss

Many population studies show that measures of body fat status are lower among those with higher physical activity levels. For example, using data from a population survey, Holcomb et al. (2004) showed that body mass index (BMI), percentage body fat, and waist-to-hip ratio each decreased with an increasing level of physical activity.

A number of meta-analyses have shown that the amount of weight lost with increases in physical activity tends to be small, and it is greater for men than for women. Ballor and Keesey (1991) conducted a meta-analysis of exercise and weight loss that included 53 studies. With an energy expenditure of nearly 1,500 kilocalories (kcal) per week from exercise for men, their mean weight loss was approximately 1.4 kilograms (kg) after approximately 16 weeks. The women had a mean energy expenditure of more than 900 kcal per week from exercise, and their mean weight loss was less than 1 kg after about 11 weeks. A similar meta-analysis by Garrow and Summerbell (1994) covering eight randomized controlled trials (five for men and three for women) found slightly greater weight loss, but the results were very similar.

Does an exercise intervention alone lead to weight loss? Studies of Targeted Risk Reduction Interventions through Defined Exercise (STRRIDE) examined this question in an 8-month randomized controlled trial of overweight untrained adults (Slentz et al., 2004). The investigators treated overweight persons with three different levels of exercise but instructed them not to change their diet. The control group gained about 1 kg; the low-amount, moderate-intensity exercise group (equivalent to walking approximately 12 miles/week) and the low-amount, vigorous-intensity exercise group (equivalent to jogging approximately 12 miles/week) lost about 1 kg. The high-amount, vigorous-intensity exercise group (equivalent to jogging approximately 20 miles/week) lost about 3.5 kg on average—4 percent of their body weight. This latter amount approaches clinical significance with regard to health benefits. Slentz et al. (2004) examined weight change per mile of exercise and estimated that covering a distance of about 6 miles/week corresponds with the amount of exercise that results in weight maintenance.

In a supervised study in which subjects came into the laboratory, Ross and colleagues (2000, 2004) found that a 500- to 700-kcal deficit per day, either through diet or exercise, produced a 6.5 percent weight loss for women and an 8 percent weight loss for men over a 12-week period.

In the 16-month, supervised Midwest Exercise Trial, Donnelly et al. (2003) found, using objective measures, that the men expended approximately 300 kcal more per session than did the women when prescribed the same relative amount of exercise in terms of frequency, intensity, and duration. With ad libitum eating, the men lost, on average, about 5 percent of their baseline weight within about 9 months. In contrast, the women did not lose weight; however, they gained little or no weight on average over the 16 months. Individual variation was substantial, especially for the women. All but one of the men in the Midwest Exercise Trial lost weight, in varying amounts, but only half of the women lost weight. As also discussed later in the session by Dr. Glenn Gaesser, other studies have produced the results illustrated in Figure 3-1.

Evidence that Physical Activity Will Benefit Weight Maintenance Among Persons Who Have Lost Weight

Qualitative evidence from the National Weight Control Registry (Klem et al., 1997) suggests that the levels of physical activity required to maintain weight following a substantial weight loss are higher than many people realize—more than 2,500 kcal/week. Weight management programs suggest that approximately 300 minutes of exercise are needed per week to produce weight maintenance for one year (LeCheminant et al., 2005).

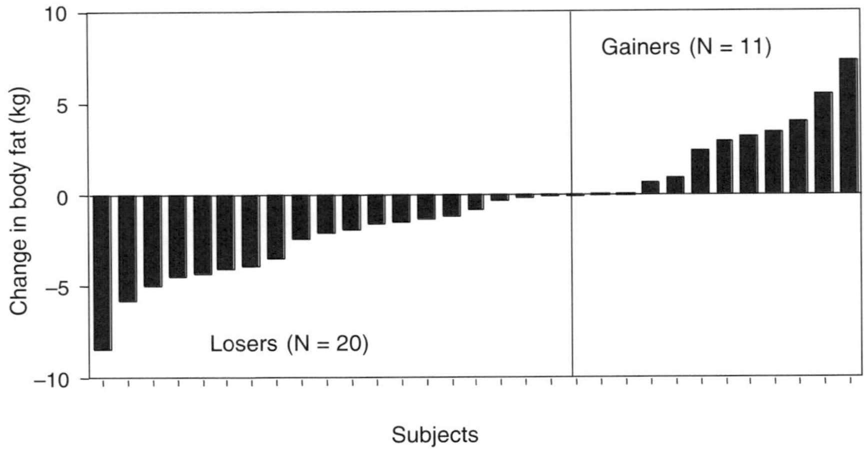

FIGURE 3-1 Individual variation in body fat mass change in response to aerobic exercise training in obese women.
SOURCE: Lamarche et al. (1992). Reprinted from *Metabolism* 41(11), Lamarche et al., Is body fat loss a determinant factor in the improvement of carbohydrate and lipid metabolism following aerobic exercise training in obese women? Pp. 1249–1256, 1992, with permission from Elsevier.

A dose–response effect was demonstrated in a study by Jakicic et al. (1999). After weight loss at 6 months, weight was maintained for 6 months by those exercising more than 200 minutes per week, whereas those exercising less than 150 minutes per week experienced regain of weight. More recent work by Jakicic and colleagues (John M. Jakicic, University of Pittsburgh, personal communication, October 16, 2006) indicates that physical activity levels were substantially higher for those who maintained a weight loss of at least 10 percent of their body weight for 18 months than for those who did not maintain that degree of weight loss.

Dr. Donnelly indicated that the randomization in most studies is done at baseline. However, randomization after weight loss is the correct study design but is rarely used. Jeffery et al. (2003) randomized subjects at baseline and at the beginning of the period of testing interventions to maintain weight. Subjects randomized to the 2,500 kcal/week exercise group maintained weight better, on average, than did those in the 1,000 kcal/week exercise group (Figure 3-2). Although there was considerable variation in exercise levels, the subjects who were asked to do more exercise did more exercise.

In a study by Borg et al. (2002) in which men were randomized after weight loss either to control or exercise groups for 6 months, a physical activity energy expenditure of approximately 2,400 kcal/week was associated with the maintenance of weight loss.

Three additional studies were found in which subjects were randomized after weight loss. In the study by Perri et al. (1988), all groups did better than the controls; but the groups assigned to behavior plus exercise did no better than the behavioral groups at 18 months. Leermakers and colleagues (1999) found that after 6 months, weight regain was lower among the exercise plus behavioral strategies group than among the group with exercise but no behavioral strategies. A somewhat confounded 24-month study by Fogelholm et al. (2000) found less weight regain among those in the 1,000 kcal/week exercise group than in the

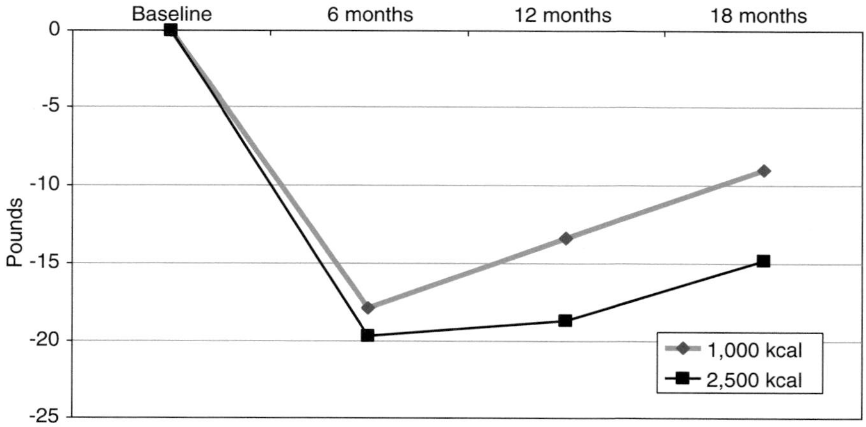

FIGURE 3-2 Mean weight change over time by treatment group.
NOTES: ♦ = standard behavior therapy (SBT) group with a goal of expending 1,000 extra kilocalories per week; ■ = high physical activity (HPA) treatment group with a goal of expending 2,500 extra kilocalories per week. SBT group marginally different from the HPA group at 12 months (p = .07) and significantly different at 18 months (p = .04).
SOURCE: Jeffery et al. (2003). Adapted, with permission, from *The American Journal of Clinical Nutrition.*

control group. There was no difference, however, between the 2,000 kcal/week exercise group and the controls, perhaps suggesting attrition problems. This suggests a benefit–risk question: Is it better to get a lower level of exercise for many years or a higher level of exercise with the risk of greater attrition?

Evidence on Physical Activity in the Prevention of Weight Gain

Dr. Donnelly presented evidence to support his position that relatively small amounts of physical activity may be sufficient to enable people to prevent unhealthy weight gain. Some investigators suggest that people gain weight in episodes related to life events such as marriage and having children, and others use a more linear perspective. Hill et al. (2003), for example, using data from the National Health and Nutrition Examination Survey and from the Coronary Artery Risk Development in Young Adults study, concluded that the energy gap for approximately 50 percent of the population may be as small as 15 kcal/day, and that specifying a gap of 50 kcal/day would cover about 90 percent of the population. Hill uses a value of 100 kcal/day to represent the energy gap, but it is acknowledged that currently there is little experimental data to support this value.

In an 18-month study with middle-aged women, Donnelly et al. (2000) showed that either 30 minutes of supervised continuous exercise three times a week or two 10- to 15-minute bouts of supervised exercise 5 days per week prevented weight gain without a dietary intervention. Dunn et al. (1999) found that sedentary men and women randomized either to lifestyle or structured exercise groups, with a goal of 1,000 kcal of energy expenditure per week, gained little or no weight in the 2-year intervention period.[1]

In an ongoing study (John M. Jakicic, University of Pittsburgh, personal communication, October 16, 2006), preliminary data show that after 18 months, subjects assigned to either 150 minutes or 300 minutes of physical activity per week weighed about 1 kilogram less than at baseline. If confirmed, this finding suggests that small amounts of physical activity may be sufficient to maintain the weight of persons who have not recently undergone a period of weight loss.

---

[1]Dr. Blair noted later that actual energy expenditure was only about 65 kcal/day.

Concluding Remarks

Physical activity or weight loss creates a relatively small energy gap and cannot be expected to provide the weight loss that is seen with energy restriction. Effects appear to differ for men and women, and there are responders and nonresponders. Dr. Donnelly took the position that the time and amount of energy expenditure required for the prevention of unhealthy weight gain appears to be 15 to 30 minutes/day or about 700 to 1,000 kcal/week. The amount of physical activity needed to achieve the loss of 5 percent of one's body weight appears to be about 45 minutes/day or 2,000 to 2,500 kcal/week. For weight-loss maintenance, the amount of physical activity required is likely to be similar to, or perhaps greater than, that for weight loss.

DISCUSSION

Aging, Inactivity, and Obesity

Discussant: Andrew Goldberg

Predictors of obesity and weight regain include high caloric intake, physical inactivity, low resting metabolic rate, low fat oxidation, reduced muscle mass, aging, decreased insulin sensitivity, and perhaps elevated adipose lipoprotein lipase activity (Ravussin and Swinburn, 1993). Aging is associated with a decline in energy expenditure, which when not compensated by a reduction in caloric intake, leads to weight gain. Regular physical activity will increase energy expenditure for older people. Maintaining energy balance with aging is critical to prevent obesity and weight regain following successful weight loss.

Studies in postmenopausal women by Goldberg and colleagues (Nicklas et al., 1996) show that weight loss, when combined with exercise training, blunts the decline in resting metabolic rate and in fat oxidation observed with weight loss alone. Dr. Goldberg's group has shown that weight loss plus an increase in VO_2max of greater than 5 percent results in several health benefits, including reductions in intra-abdominal fat and insulin resistance; improvements in glucose tolerance, insulin sensitivity, and blood pressure; reductions in total and low density lipoprotein cholesterol and triglycerides; and increases in high density lipoprotein cholesterol (Lynch et al., 2001).

A study by Bunyard et al. (1998) shows that both obese and lean sedentary middle-aged men were able to increase their exercise capacity by 15 percent with an aerobic exercise program. The lean sedentary group lost about 1.8 kg after 6 months of training despite increasing their caloric intake, and the obese sedentary men lost about 8 kg after 6 months of the exercise training plus hypocaloric weight loss instruction. Master athletes who discontinued exercise training for 8 weeks experienced a reduction in VO_2max of about 15 percent and gained about 0.5 kg, despite reducing their caloric intake by 17 percent. All groups converged to about the same level of fitness, but when placed on isocaloric weight maintaining diets, the obese and lean men were able to consume 5 percent and 8 percent more calories, respectively, without gaining weight. These results provide evidence that sedentary older people can change their daily exercise habits to increase their energy expenditure from physical activity, allowing them to eat more without gaining weight. Thus regular aerobic exercise, by increasing daily energy expenditure, may counter the age-related tendency toward obesity and its associated cardiovascular risk factors.

Preliminary studies are in progress in Dr. Goldberg's laboratory to test the hypothesis that weight loss, when combined with aerobic exercise training, will maintain both the resting metabolic rate and the oxidation of fat and carbohydrate, with subsequent cardiometabolic and weight maintenance benefits (Ortmeyer et al., 2006). This hypothesis is illustrated in Figure 3-3. Our understanding of the potential benefits of exercise training for weight management in obese middle-aged and older people may be enhanced by knowledge of the metabolic mechanisms by which exercise, when combined with weight loss, increases fat and carbohydrate oxidation in muscle.

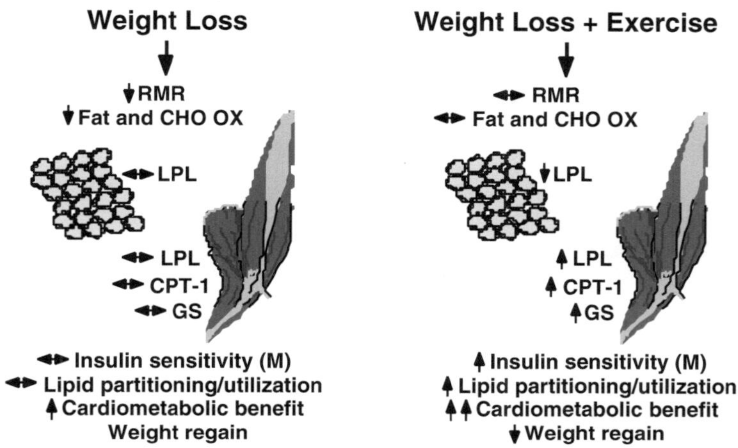

FIGURE 3-3 Hypothesis: Metabolic adaptations to weight loss with or without aerobic exercise.
NOTE: RMR=resting metabolic rate; CHO=carbohydrate; OX=oxidation; LPL=lipoprotein lipase; CPT-1=carnitine palmitoyltransferase-1; GS=glycogen synthase.
SOURCE: Goldberg (2006).

Additional Epidemiological Data on Physical Activity and Weight

Discussant: Glenn Gaesser

As the prevalence of obesity has risen, so have weight loss attempts—without much apparent success. Epidemiological studies of women and men in the United States indicate a tendency for an inverse relationship between BMI and physical activity (Feskanich et al., 2002; Hu et al., 1999; Kushi et al., 1997). Studies in a number of other countries show mixed findings, with most showing an inverse relationship between BMI and physical activity for men (Andersen et al., 2000; Hu et al., 2003; Rosengren and Wilhemsen, 1997; Thune et al., 1998) and women (Andersen et al., 2000; Hu et al., 2003; Mensink et al., 1999). However, some studies show no relationship for men (Bijnen et al., 1998; Smith et al., 2000) or for women (Thune et al., 1998). In studies reporting the strongest inverse associations between BMI and physical activity, the mean BMI is no more than one to two BMI units lower for those at a high physical activity level than for those at a low physical activity level (Feskanich et al., 2002; Hu et al., 1999, 2003; Kushi et al., 1997).

Data from Rosell et al. (2006) indicate that weight gain tended to be modestly less for more active than for less active persons over a 5-year period. Petrella et al. (2005) reported similar findings of a modest benefit of physical activity over a 10-year period among older persons. Notably, compared to weight change in younger persons, change in weight tends to be of smaller magnitude in older individuals.

Larmarche et al. (1992) demonstrated that, among obese women who participated in exercise training, both those who lost fat and those who gained fat had improvements in VO_2max, glucose tolerance, and blood lipid concentrations. Thus, regardless of the response measured by weight change or body fat change, individuals in the exercise program responded favorably in terms of indicators of health. Earlier work by Bjorntorp et al. (1970) found improvement in insulin sensitivity after exercise training with an *increase* in body fat.

In summary, cohort studies reveal an inverse association between physical activity and BMI, but the effect is relatively small. Physical activity may be more effective in preventing unhealthy weight gain than in producing weight loss. Many weight-related health problems can be improved with exercise independently of weight loss. This latter point merits emphasis in view of the very modest effect of exercise on inducing weight change in women.

Group Discussion

Moderator: Peter Brubaker

During the group discussion, workshop presenters and other participants raised the following points:

- Walking and running the same distance are not actually equivalent in energy expenditure. Several persons suggested that pointing out the discrepancy would be counterproductive because the concept is difficult to understand.
- Despite the modest effect of physical activity on weight loss, certain health benefits do not occur without a physical activity component of treatment.

- Maintenance of healthy weight when children are growing is a very important focus. Factors involved include physical education programs, allowed recess activities, extracurricular activities, and potentially, short bouts of physical activity in the classroom.
- Research in older disabled people has found that a moderate increase in VO_2max leads to marked improvements in glucose metabolism, insulin levels, and glucose tolerance, implying benefit for older people in general.

REFERENCES

Andersen LB, Schnohr P, Schroll M, Hein MO. 2000. All-cause mortality associated with physical activity during leisure time, work, sports, and cycling to work. *Arch Intern Med* 160(11):1621–1628.

Ballor DL, and Keesey RE. 1991. A meta-analysis of the factors affecting exercise-induced changes in body mass, fat mass, and fat-free mass in males and females. *Int J Obes* 15(11):717–726.

Bijnen FCH, Casperson CJ, Feskins EJM, Saris WHM, Mosterd WL, Kromhout D. 1998. Physical activity and 10-year mortality from cardiovascular disease. *Arch Intern Med* 158(14):1499–1505.

Bjorntorp P, De Jounge K, Sjostrom L, Sullivan L. 1970. The effect of physical training on insulin production in obesity. *Metabolism* 19(8):631–638.

Borg P, Kukkonen-Harjula K, Fogelholm M, Pasanen M. 2002. Effects of walking or resistance training on weight loss maintenance in obese, middle-aged men: A randomized trial. *Int J Obesity* 26(5):676–683.

Bunyard LB, Katzel LI, Busby-Whitehead MJ, Wu Z, Goldberg AP. 1998. Energy requirements of middle-aged men are modifiable by physical activity. *Am J Clin Nutr* 68(5):1136–1142.

Donnelly JE, Jacobsen DJ, Snyder Heelan KA, Seip R, Smith S. 2000. The effects of 18 months of intermittent vs continuous exercise on aerobic capacity, body weight and composition, and metabolic fitness in previously sedentary, moderately obese females. *Int J Obes* 24(5):566–572.

Donnelly JE, Hill JO, Jacobsen DJ, Potteiger J, Sullivan DK, Johnson SL, Heelan K, Hise M, Fennessey PV, Sonko B, Sharp T, Jakicic JM, Blair SN, Tran ZV, Mayo M, Gibson C, Washburn RA. 2003. Effects of a 16-month randomized controlled exercise trial on body weight and composition in young, overweight men and women: The Midwest Exercise Trial (MET). *Arch Intern Med* 163(11):1343–1350.

Dunn AL, Marcus BH, Kampert JB, Garcia ME, Kohl HW, Brasel JA. 1999. Comparison of lifestyle and structured interventions to increase physical activity and cardiorespiratory fitness. *J Am Med Assoc* 281(4):327–334.

Feskanich D, Willett W, Colditz G. 2002. Walking and leisure-time activity and risk of hip fracture in postmenopausal women. *J Am Med Assoc* 288(18):2300–2306.

Fogelholm M, Kukkonen-Harjula K, Nenonen A, Pasanen M. 2000. Effects of walking training on weight maintenance after a very-low-energy diet in premenopausal obese women: A randomized controlled trial. *Arch Intern Med* 160(14):2177–2184.

Garrow J, Summerbell C. 1994. Meta analysis on the effect of exercise on the composition of weight loss. *Int J Obes* 18(7):516-517.

Goldberg AP. 2006. Presentation at the Institute of Medicine Physical Activity Guidelines Development Workshop. Washington, DC. October 23.

Hill JO, Wyatt HR, Reed GW, Peters JC. 2003. Obesity and the environment: Where do we go from here? *Science* 299(5608):853–855.

Holcomb CA, Heim DL, Loughin TM. 2004. Physical activity minimizes the association of body fatness with abdominal obesity in white, premenopausal women: Results from the Third National Health and Nutrition Examination Survey. *J Am Diet Assoc* 104(12):1859–1862.

Hu FB, Sigal RJ, Rich-Edwards JW, Colditz GA, Solomon CG, Willett WC, Speizer FE, Manson JE. 1999. Walking compared with vigorous physical activity and risk of type 2 diabetes in women: A prospective study. *J Am Med Assoc* 282(15):1433–1439.

Hu G, Qiao Q, Silventoinen K, Eriksson JG, Jousilahti P, Lindstrom J, Valle TT, Nissinen A, Tuomilehto J. 2003. Occupational, commuting, and leisure-time physical activity in relation to risk for type 2 diabetes in middle-aged Finnish men and women. *Diabetologia* 46(3):322–329.

Jakicic JM, Winters C, Lang W, Wing RR. 1999. Effects of intermittent exercise and use of home exercise equipment on adherence, weight loss, and fitness in overweight women. *J Am Med Assoc* 282(16):1554–1560.

Jeffery RW, Wing RR, Sherwood NE, Tata DF. 2003. Physical activity and weight loss: Does prescribing higher physical activity goals improve outcome? *Am J Clin Nutr* 78(4):684–689.

Klem ML, Wing RR, McGuire MT, Seagle HM, Hill JO. 1997. A descriptive study of individuals successful at long-term maintenance of substantial weight loss. *Am J Clin Nutr* 66(2):239–246.

Kushi LH, Fee RM, Folsom AR, Mink PJ, Anderson KE, Sellers TA. 1997. Physical activity and mortality in postmenopausal women. *J Am Med Assoc* 277(16):1287–1292.

Lamarche B, Despres JP, Pouliot MC, Moorjani S, Lupien PJ, Theriault G, Tremblay A, Nadeau A, Bouchard C. 1992. Is body fat loss a determinant factor in the improvement of carbohydrate and lipid metabolism following aerobic exercise training in obese women? *Metabolism* 41(11):1249–1256.

LeCheminant JD, Jacobsen DJ, Hall MA, Donnelly JE. 2005. A comparison of meal replacements and medication in weight maintenance after weight loss. *Am J Clin Nutr* 24(5):347–353.

Leermakers EA, Perri MG, Shigaki CL, Fuller PR. 1999. Effects of exercise-focused versus weight-focused maintenance programs on the management of obesity. *Addict Behav* 24(2):219–227.

Lynch NA, Nicklas BJ, Berman DM, Dennis KE, Goldberg AP. 2001. Reductions in visceral fat during weight loss and walking are associated with improvements in VO_2max. *J Appl Physiol* 90(1):99–104.

Mensink GBM, Ziese T, Kok FJ. 1999. Benefits of leisure-time physical activity on the cardiovascular risk profile at older age. *Int J Epidemiol* 28(4):659–666.

Nicklas BJ, Rogus EM, Colman EG, Goldberg AP. 1996. Visceral adiposity, increased adipocyte lipolysis, and metabolic dysfunction in obese postmenopausal women. *Am J Physiol* 33(1):E72–E78.

Ortmeyer HK, Ryan AS, Blumenthal JB, Joseph LJO, Goldberg AP. 2006. Exercise and weight loss (WL), but not WL alone, affects skeletal muscle and adipose tissue lipoprotein lipase activity in post-menopausal women. *Diabetes* 55(Suppl 1):A5.

Perri MG, McAllister DA, Gange JJ, Jordan RC, McAdoo G, and Nezu AM. 1988. Effects of four maintenance programs on the long-term management of obesity. *J Consult Clin Psychol* 56(4):529–534.

Petrella RJ, Lattanzio CN, Demeray A, Varallo V, Blore R. 2005. Can adoption of regular exercise later in life prevent metabolic risk for cardiovascular disease? *Diabetes Care* 28(3):694–701.

Ravussin E, Swinburn BA. 1993. Metabolic predictors of obesity: Cross-sectional versus longitudinal data. *Int J Obes* 17(Suppl 3):S28–S31.

Rosell M, Appleby P, Spencer E, Key T. 2006. Weight gain over 5 years in 21 966 meat-eating, fish-eating, vegetarian, and vegan men and women in EPIC-Oxford. *Int J Obes* 30(9):1389–1396.

Rosengren A, Wilhelmsen L. 1997. Physical activity protects against coronary death and deaths from all causes in middle-aged men. *Ann Epidemiol* 7(1): 69–75.

Ross R, Dagnone D, Jones PJ, Smith H, Paddags A, Hudson R, and Janssen I. 2000. Reduction in obesity and related comorbid conditions after diet-induced weight loss or exercise-induced weight loss in men. A randomized, controlled trial. *Ann Intern Med* 133(2):92–103.

Ross R, Janssen I, Dawson J, Kungl AM, Kuk JL, Wong SL, Nguyen-Duy TB, Lee S, Kilpatrick K, and Hudson R. 2004. Exercise-induced reduction in obesity and insulin resistance in women: A randomized controlled trial. *Obes Res* 12(5):789–798.

Slentz CA, Duscha BD, Johnson JL, Ketchum K, Aiken LB, Samsa GP, Houmard JA, Bales CW, and Kraus WE. 2004. Effects of the amount of exercise on body weight, body composition, and measures of central obesity: STRRIDE—a randomized controlled study. *Arch Intern Med* 164(1):31–39.

Smith GD, Shipley MJ, Batty GD, Morris JN, Marmot M. 2000. Physical activity and cause-specific mortality in the Whitehall study. *Public Health* 114(5):308–315.

Thune I, Njolstad I, Lochen M-L, Forde OH. 1998. Physical activity improves the metabolic risk profiles in men and women. The Tromso Study. *Arch Intern Med* 158(15):1633–1640.

4

Physical Activity and Risk—Maximizing Benefits

Physical activity can pose risks in two main areas: musculoskeletal injury and fatal and nonfatal cardiac events. This chapter first addresses injury risk and then cardiovascular risk. Both sections of the chapter include evidence regarding reduction of the risk. The discussion section provides an overview of risk–benefit considerations and of osteoarthritis and joint injuries in relation to physical activity, and it offers a brief summary of comments raised by the workshop participants.

RISKS OF MUSCULOSKELETAL INJURY

Presenter: Bruce H. Jones[1]

This presentation included background information about risks and the incidence of musculoskeletal injury, a summary of factors affecting risks of injuries, and a summary of key conclusions about the causes, risk factors, and prevention of physical activity-related injury.

Background

In 1984, the Centers for Disease Control[2] held a workshop on the public health aspects of physical activity. Injuries were identified as a risk about which limited information was available (Koplan et al., 1985).

---

[1]Dr. Jones acknowledged assistance from Dr. Joseph Knapik.
[2]Renamed the Centers for Disease Control and Prevention in 1992.

To help prevent injuries related to physical activity, answers to the following questions are needed:

- How big is the problem?
- What causes the problem?
- Are there modifiable risk factors?
- What works to prevent the problem?

To answer these questions, it is useful to focus on the evidence for weight-bearing physical activity—the injury problem that has been most studied. Data are available from studies of runners, walkers, and military trainees.

Self-reported injury rates (counting both overuse and trauma) have been estimated to be between 25 to 65 injuries per 100 person-years for runners (Jones et al., 1994), 42 per 100 person-years for walkers (Suter et al., 1994), and 110 per 100 person-years for cyclists (Wilbur et al., 1995). Injury rates from studies based on routine clinical follow-up or medical records are much higher for activities such as aerobic dance (Garrick et al., 1986), exercise and recreational sports (Requa et al., 1993), and army basic training (Jones et al, 1994). Thus injury can be a substantial problem for a variety of exercise groups.

Factors Affecting the Risk of Injury

The factors that affect the risk of physical activity-related injury include the amount and type of current physical activity, the amount of past physical activity, other health behaviors, physical fitness level, history of previous injury, selected demographic factors, and anatomical factors.

Current Physical Activity

Amount of physical activity The risk of injury increases as the distance run per week increases (Koplan et al., 1982). However, the injury risk per 100 kilometers run decreases with an increase in the number of kilometers run per week (Jones et al., 1994). A number of studies confirm that greater amounts[3] of running result in higher rates of injury among civilian runners (Brunet et al., 1990; Colbert et al., 2000; Macera et al., 1989; Marti et al., 1988; Walter et al., 1989) and among military recruits (Almeida et al., 1999). For walking, the risks of injury are similar over the range of less than 15 minutes of walking per day to more than 30 minutes per day (Colbert et al., 2000).

For previously sedentary individuals exercising three days per week, a threshold for elevated injury risk appeared between about 30 and 45 minutes per day of running (Pollock et al., 1977). That is, injury risk more than doubled, whereas endurance improved little or not at all. A study of army trainees showed a similar threshold of elevated injury risk with no gain in aerobic fitness at between 5 and 10 miles of running per week (Jones et al., 1994).

Type of physical activity Few studies allow the comparison of different types of activities using the same definitions of injury and the same measures of exposure. Hootman and colleagues (2001), however, provide useful data (Table 4-1). Notably, sedentary individuals have about a 15 percent risk of injury. By comparison, walkers are at only slightly higher risk than sedentary people, while runners and those involved in sports (especially men) are at substantially higher risk.

TABLE 4-1 Injury[a] Risks Among Men and Women by Type of Physical Activity

Type of Activity (Number of Subjects)	Risk by Sex, percent per year (relative risk)	
	Men	Women
Sedentary (1,608 M, 501 W)	14.6[b] (1.0)	16.8[b] (1.0)
Walking (508 M, 206 W)	16.5 (1.14)	19.9 (1.18)
Running (2,445 M, 405 W)	24.7 (1.78)	23.2 (1.38)
Sports (467 M, 101 W)	27.6 (1.89)	26.7 (1.59)

NOTE: M = men, W = women.
[a]Self-reported injury in the previous year.
[b]Significantly lower than all activities, Chi squared $p < .05$.
SOURCE: Adapted from Hootman et al. (2001).

[3]Amount refers to duration x frequency x intensity.

Past Physical Activity

Five well-designed studies report that greater frequency or duration of past physical activity is associated with a lower risk of current injury (Jones et al., 1993b; Knapik et al., 2001; Rauh et al., 2006b; Shaffer et al., 1999, 2006). Among male U.S. Army trainees, for example, those who ran at least 4 days per week the month before initial entry training had a 20 percent risk of injury, whereas those who ran 3 or fewer days per week had about twice the risk. Similar results are reported for other types of exercise.

Physical Fitness Levels

Health-related components of fitness include endurance, muscle endurance, muscle strength, flexibility, and body composition (Caspersen et al., 1985). A very consistent finding in the military studies is that the more aerobically fit a person is, the lower the incidence of injury (Jones et al., 1993a; Knapik et al., 1993, 1998, 2001; Rauh et al., 2006b; Reynolds et al., 1994; Shaffer et al., 2006).

Data on improvement in 2-mile run times among army recruits shows that the trainees in the slowest quartile of trainees reduce their time by an average of 5.5 minutes while the trainees in the fastest quartile reduce their time by an average of 1.1 minutes (Knapik et al., 2006). Data such as these suggest that the least aerobically fit trainees on entry to the service may move themselves into a lower risk category and reduce their risk of injury by 30 to 50 percent over the current 9-week period of basic training.

Data on civilian populations suggests the opposite effect from military trainees, that the most fit civilians may be at highest risk (Hootman et al., 2001). It has been suggested that the most fit runners and exercise participants may place themselves at higher risk because they do more exercise at higher intensities than their less fit peers (Hootman et al., 2001).

Associations of other health-related components of fitness with injury vary:

- Compared with aerobic fitness, the muscle endurance of military personnel shows similar association to injury risk, but the reported associations are weaker (Bell et al., 2000; Jones et al., 1993b, 1994; Knapik et al., 1998, 2001).

- Muscle strength shows inconsistent association with injury risk (Jones et al., 1993b; Knapik et al., 2001; Westphal et al., 1995).
- Flexibility has a bimodal association with injury risk (Jones et al., 1993b; Knapik et al., 1992, 2001). Those who are loose (most flexible) and those who are tight (least flexible) have the highest incidence of physical activity injury, which is about twice as high as those of average flexibility.
- Body composition has inconsistent associations with injury risk (Hootman et al., 2001; Jones et al., 1992, 1993a; Macera et al., 1989; Reynolds et al., 1994; Taunton et al., 2003). When fitness data are stratified by body mass index, it appears that the leanest, slowest individuals are at greatest risk for injury (NRC, 2006).

Health and Health Behaviors

Among the common health and health behavior risk factors for physical injury are:

- past injury (Hootman et al., 2001; Jones et al., 1993b; Macera et al., 1989; Walter et al., 1989),
- amenorrhea (Barrow and Saha, 1988; Lloyd et al., 1986; Rauh et al., 2006b; Shaffer et al., 2006),
- sedentary lifestyle (Gardner et al., 1988; Jones et al., 1992, 1993b; Knapik et al., 2001), and
- cigarette smoking (Altarac et al., 2000; Jones et al., 1993b; Knapik et al., 2001; Reynolds et al., 1994).

Selected Demographic Factors

Age Studies of associations of older age with the risk of injury have produced inconsistent results. Eight studies indicate that older age is associated with higher risk of injury (Brudvig et al., 1983; Gardner et al., 1988; Jones et al., 1993b; Knapik et al., 2001, 2006; McKean et al., 2006; Shaffer et al., 1999; Taunton et al., 2003). Four studies show that older age is associated with lower risk (Carlson et al., 2006; Colbert et al., 2000; Hootman et al., 2001; Knapik et al., 1993). Most of the studies that show higher risk with older age are military studies. It may be that older civilian exercise participants modulate their risk of injury by performing less exercise at lower intensities.

Sex During army basic training where male and female trainees do the same physical training, females are at 1.6 to 2.1 times greater risk for injury than males (Bell et al., 2000; Bensel et al., 1983; Canham et al., 1998; Jones et al., 1992; Knapik et al., 2003; Kowal, 1980). After adjusting for physical fitness (Canham et al., 1998)—or for physical fitness, age, and race (Bell et al., 2000)—the risk is essentially the same.

Anatomical Factors

Some anatomical factors (e.g., foot morphology, knee Q-angle) appear to be associated with the risk of injury (Brunet et al., 1990; Cowan et al., 1994, 1996; Giladi et al., 1985; Rauh et al., 2006a), but such factors may not be amenable to correction. Evidence indicates that bone, muscle, tendons, and ligaments adapt to increased physical activity and exercise (Maffulli and King, 1992; Maganaris et al., 2004; Sharma and Maffulli, 2006). Structured regimens to improve the resistance of these tissues to injury have not yet been tested.

Evidence for the Prevention of Weight-Bearing Physical Activity-Related Injuries

In 2003, a new standardized program to prevent over-training during army basic training found that the traditional physical training program posed a significantly higher risk than did the injury prevention program (Knapik et al., 2004b, 2005). Features of the standardized injury prevention program include reduced miles run, performance of distance runs by ability groups, the addition of speed drills, and a more balanced program of activities. Other trials of similar methods have been successful (Knapik et al., 2003, 2004a; Rudzki and Cunningham, 1999; Shaffer et al., 1996). Other prevention strategies appear to have a limited effect or no effect on reducing risk. These other strategies include stretching (Herbert and Gabriel, 2002; Rome et al., 2005; Shrier,1999; Thacker et al., 2004), warm-ups (Fradkin et al., 2006), and shock absorbent devices for footwear (D'hondt et al., 2002/2005; Jones et al., 2002; Rome et al., 2005; Withnall et al., 2006; Yeung and Yeung, 2001).

Concluding Remarks

Greater amounts of physical activity increase the risk of injury, and thresholds of physical activity exist above which more activity increases injury risk but not fitness. More past physical activity and higher fitness levels protect against injuries. In addition to lack of fitness, modifiable risks include amenorrhea, inactivity, and smoking. The prevention of overtraining can reduce injury risk and improve fitness. Dr. Jones expressed the view that (1) sufficient evidence is available to establish general principles of physical activity-related injury causation and prevention, and (2) the application of those principles is expected to maximize the benefits and minimize the risks of physical activity.

PHYSICAL ACTIVITY AND CARDIOVASCULAR DISEASE RISKS

Presenter: David S. Siscovick

The primary focus of this presentation was on sudden cardiac arrest among individuals older than about 30 years, with some attention to nonfatal myocardial infarction. Because the overall effect of exercise on cardiovascular health reflects a potential balance of benefits and risks, the presentation included a review of evidence regarding the magnitude of risk, factors that modify risk, data on the balance of the risks and benefits, and implications for public health and for clinical care.

Magnitude of the Problem

About 10 to 15 percent of all deaths from coronary heart disease are due to sudden cardiac arrest. Approximately 5 percent of cardiac arrests occur during vigorous exercise, and about 10 percent of cardiac arrests occur during moderate-intensity exercise. The magnitude of the risk varies with the nature of the physical activity, the environment, characteristics of the population, and other factors. Reported values for absolute risk per exerciser range from 1 cardiac arrest in 5,000 individuals per year at an aerobics center to 1 in 20,000 individuals per year in the general population during vigorous activity. Examined in a different way, the ratio of the risk during the activity compared to the risk at other times ranged from 4.5 for cross-country skiing in Finland to 7 for joggers in Rhode Island.

Factors that Modify Risk

Factors that modify the risk of cardiac arrest during exercise can be organized by characteristics of the exercise, characteristics of the exerciser, environmental factors, and personal habits. Little evidence is available about the impact of environmental factors (temperature, humidity, altitude, air pollution) or about the impact of personal habits (such as the use of alcohol or tobacco) on the risk of cardiac arrest during exercise. Thus Dr. Siscovick focused on characteristics of the exercise and of the exerciser.

Characteristics of the Exercise

Both the intensity of the exercise and the habitual level of physical activity can affect the risk of cardiac arrest. In a large study in Finland, Vuori (1986) showed that there was a 9-fold increase in the risk of having a sudden cardiac arrest during vigorous exercise compared to other times and a 3.2-fold increase in risk during nonvigorous exercise. To examine the risks of the exercise in relation to the potential benefits of physical activity, Siscovick and colleagues (1984) collected data on the type, intensity, frequency, and duration of activity; and then they estimated the time spent on activity to examine the risks, both during and not during activity, in terms of incidence density.

Characteristics that Modify Absolute Risk

Clinical heart disease In the presence of clinical heart disease, both the risk during activity and the risk not during activity are increased. However, the magnitude of the increase in risk during activity compared to not during activity is about seven-fold (Siscovick, 1997). This is similar to that for the general population.

Sex The absolute risk of sudden cardiac arrest overall and during bouts of moderate to vigorous exertion are much lower in women than in men, as is the relative risk. During moderate or vigorous exertion by women, the absolute risk of sudden cardiac arrest increased about two-fold, compared to other times, but the magnitude of the risk was very much lower than that in men (Whang et al., 2006). As with men, the training or habitual activity level was associated with a lower risk during a bout of moderate to intense exertion.

Age Data from Vuori (1986) indicate that the *absolute* risk of sudden death during exercise increases with age, but sudden death is very uncommon among persons younger than 45 years. The *relative* risk of sudden cardiac arrest during vigorous exercise compared to other times is much higher in men younger than 45 years than in older men because the absolute risk of sudden cardiac arrest that occurs during inactivity is very low in younger men.

Habitual physical activity The data in Table 4-2 indicate that the magnitude of the transient increase in risk during exercise was influenced by the level of habitual vigorous exercise. The increase in risk during exercise was lowest among the men who were engaged in more than 124 kilocalories (kcal) (20 minutes) of vigorous exercise per day. The impact of habitual activity on the transient increase in risk during a bout of activity is consistent with a training effect, possibly due to reduced physiological and metabolic stress among men who engage in habitual vigorous exercise.

Some years later, Albert et al. (2000) reported similar findings using data from the Physicians' Health Study. The overall occurrence of sudden death during vigorous exercise was very small. However, the evidence suggested a much greater risk of having a sudden cardiac arrest during vigorous exertion among the physicians who exercised less than once per week than among those who exercised at least five times per week. These investigators also examined the data to look for a circadian variation in the risk of exertion, but they found no difference in the transient increase in risk during vigorous exertion occurring in the morning, afternoon, or at night.

TABLE 4-2 Sudden Cardiac Arrest During Vigorous Exercise: Balance of Cardiac Risk and Benefits

	Cases/10^8 Person Hours (N)		
Habitual Vigorous Exercise, kcal/day	During Activity	Not During Activity	Overall[a]
0	NA	18 (30)	18 (34)
1–16	732 (2)	13 (44)	14 (46)
17–123	66 (3)	5 (32)	6 (35)
>124	21 (4)	4 (10	5 (22)

NOTE: 10^8 = 100 million.
[a]The weighted average of the risk during and not during exercise in which the weights are the amount of time spent in exercise.
SOURCE: Siscovick et al. (1984).

Looking at vigorous exertion as a potential trigger of acute nonfatal myocardial infarction, Mittleman et al. (1993) demonstrated that a transient increase in the risk of a nonfatal myocardial infarction occurs within the hour after a bout of vigorous exertion. As with the investigators above who examined increases in the risk of sudden cardiac arrest, Mittleman and colleagues (1993) found that the relative risk of nonfatal myocardial infarction for heavy exertion decreased dramatically with increased frequency of regular physical exertion, reported as numbers of bouts per week.

Balance of Cardiac Risks and Benefits

The data in column 4 of Table 4-2 also indicate that the overall incidence of sudden cardiac arrest (the weighted average of the risk during and not during exercise where the weights are the amount of time spent in exercise) was highest among those who did not engage in habitual vigorous exercise. With increasing levels of habitual activity, the overall risk of sudden cardiac arrest decreases substantially, despite the transient increase in risk during activity compared to the risk at other times. Physical activity can be compared to surgery—similar to surgery, physical activity poses acute risks, but it also has the potential for supporting a longer, healthier life.

Limitations of the Available Evidence

Several limitations of the available evidence need to be considered. There is a lack of consistency in the definition of cardiac events during exertion. Specifically, some investigators define events within 30 to 60 minutes of a bout of exertion as "during exertion." In addition, most studies have only a small number of events during exertion. In general, there is a lack of detail about prior habitual activity and the presence of prior heart disease and coronary risk factors, and current data are not yet sufficient to predict cardiac events during exertion.

Concluding Remarks

Dr. Siscovick presented his assessment of public health implications and clinical implications as follows:

Public Health Implications

Exercise has acute cardiac risks, but the absolute risk of a cardiac event during exercise is low, and the transient increase in risk is outweighed by the long-term cardiac benefits of exercise. A number of factors modify risk. In advising the public, it is important to consider both risks and benefits.

Clinical Implications

When providing clinical care, an important measure is targeting exercise, and considering environmental factors and habits. This requires asking patients about the circumstances under which they exercise. In part because the sensitivity of pre-exercise evaluation is low in adults, medical supervision of exercise is indicated for selected individuals (such as those with clinical coronary heart disease). Automated external defibrillators in settings of supervised exercise may be very helpful in resuscitating individuals who have a cardiac arrest.

DISCUSSION

Physical Activity-Related Injuries: Is the Benefit Worth the Risk?

Discussant: Jennifer Hootman

Risk Associated with Physical Activity

Among civilian, community-dwelling adults in the United States, the incidence of physical activity-related injury is very low overall, but it ranges widely for specific groups (for example, the range is 8 to 80 percent for recreational and competitive runners). The more active a person is, the higher the probability of injury (Hootman et al., 2002; Pollock et al., 1977). Nonetheless, about 15 percent of sedentary people report an activity-related injury. As indicated earlier by Dr. Jones, with increases in activity, the risk per unit of exercise exposure may be lower.

Using unadjusted data, Hootman and colleagues found that people who meet the Surgeon General's physical activity recommendation (defined as 1,000 kcal or more of physical activity-related energy expenditure per week) have a risk of injury that is about 77 percent higher than that of inactive people (zero energy expenditure from physical activity per week). After adjusting for a variety of risk factors (mainly the modifiable risk factors identified by Dr. Jones), however, the increase in risk is not statistically significant for both men and women. The results of a multivariate analysis suggest that (1) even insufficient exercise (1 to 999 kcal of exercise per week) may confer a small amount of protection against activity-related injury, and (2) twice weekly weight training and stretching exercise each may also confer a small amount of protection against activity-related injury.

A few studies report injury rates per 1,000 hours of physical activity. Reported rates include 0.19 to 1.5 for commuting and lifestyle activities (Parkkari et al., 2004), 2.2 for strength and aerobic exercise in older adults (Colbert et al., 2000), 5.9 to 7.8 for adult fitness activities (Requa et al., 1993), and 6.6 to 18.3 for recreational sports (Parkkari et al., 2004). According to Dr. Hootman, the injury rate can be estimated to be about one injury every 4 years for the average person who meets the minimal public health recommendation for physical activity. The basis for the estimate is in Box 4-1.

BOX 4-1

Estimation of Injury Rate for Individuals Meeting the Surgeon General's Physical Activity Recommendation

Physical activity recommendation = 30 minutes of exercise 5 days/week.

- 150 minutes/week =
- 7,800 minutes or 130 hours/year =
- 7.7 years to accumulate 1,000 hours of activity

If the injury rate is approximately 2.0/1,000 hours, then the injury rate is about one injury every 4 years.

SOURCE: Colbert et al. (2000).

Possible Prevention Messages

Dr. Hootman listed a number of possible prevention messages and the type of evidence that supports each, as follows:

- Choose activities wisely. Walking poses 50 percent less risk than does running.
- Moderate the total dose of physical activity. Exercising more than 20 miles per week increases the risk 1.7 to 2.1 times.
- Combine strengthening with aerobic exercise. Strength training reduces the risk about 40 percent in women.
- Maintain a normal body weight. Although it is not known if weight loss reduces the risk of injury, it improves biomechanics.
- Improve fitness level slowly before entering a rigorous training program. Military data show the importance of this approach.
- Obtain appropriate care and rehabilitation before returning to participation post injury. Previous injury is a risk factor for a future injury.

Concluding Remarks

Dr. Hootman expressed the view that the benefits do outweigh the risks and that there are ways to modify the risks.

Physical Activity, Osteoarthritis, and Joint Injuries

Discussant: William E. Garrett, Jr.

In his discussion, Dr. Garrett focused on the potential association between exercise and osteoarthritis (OA) rather than on a single injury. Among the many reasons people provide for not exercising are the association between exercise and pain and the understandable concern that exercise-related pain could lead to OA. Although OA has been linked to "wear and tear," some evidence suggests that exercise that promotes muscle strength and endurance may allow the muscles rather than the bones and joints to absorb the energy preferentially. By this concept, exercise may even protect from OA (Hurley, 1999; Shrier et al., 2004). Diseases such as diabetes lead to muscle weakness and sensory neuropathy that can cause extreme arthritis in the form of Charcot joints—even with very little exercise.

The clear associations between exercise and OA involve sports (e.g., soccer, football, and basketball) that may lead to joint injury such as ligament or meniscal damage in the knee. Data are unclear regarding whether there is an association between running and OA, but moderate levels of running or of other aerobic exercise do not appear to cause OA (Konradsen et al., 1990; White et al., 1993). Professional groups such as the American College of Rheumatology include aerobic and strengthening exercises in the treatment of people with OA.

Joint Injuries

Relatively high rates of joint injuries occur in sports. These injuries can lead to changes of OA and are a better predictor of OA than sports participation itself (Thelin et al., 2006). The development and implementation of injury prevention programs could help achieve the benefits of exercise without the risk of OA.

Concluding Remarks

Given all the health benefits of exercise and the lack of an association between exercise and OA, health care professionals can provide a useful service by prescribing exercise regularly and alleviating patient concerns regarding arthritis.

Group Discussion

Moderator: Caroline Macera

Points raised during the group discussion included the following:

- Few data are available regarding traumatic injury risk associated with exercise such as running, racing, and bicycling.
- Data are needed regarding physical activity-related injury in the context of all injury. For example, can physical activity provide protection from other types of injuries?
- Definitions related to injury need to be standardized. In general, the injuries that are counted are those that require some medical treatment and result in a change in activity level.
- The primary cause of sudden cardiac death among U.S. adults is coronary heart disease. Risk factors for coronary heart disease are likely to increase the risk of sudden cardiac death both during activity and during inactivity. For persons with previously expressed cardiovascular disease, a supervised setting for exercise is beneficial.
- Screening guidelines for the general population and those with cardiovascular risk factors need clarification. Results of submaximal tests on middle-aged men with elevated low-density lipoprotein cholesterol concentration have low sensitivity.
- Findings from the Wisconsin Epidemiological Study on Diabetic Retinopathy related to weight lifting may provide useful information on adverse effects of physical activity on microvascular disease.
- An article by Carato and a review by Thompson (2005) provide potentially useful information about cardiovascular events during exercise among athletes and the potential impact of pre-exercise evaluations among young people.

REFERENCES

Albert CM, Mitleman MA, Chae CU, Lee IM, Hennekens CH, Manson JE. 2000. Triggering of sudden death from cardiac causes by vigorous exertion. *N Engl J Med* 343(19):1355–1361.

Almeida SA, Williams KM, Shaffer RA, Brodine SK. 1999. Epidemiological patterns of musculoskeletal injuries and physical training. *Med Sci Sports Exerc* 31(8):1176–1182.

Altarac M, Gardner JW, Popovich RM, Potter R, Knapik JJ, Jones BH. 2000. Cigarette smoking and exercise-related injuries among young men and women. *Am J Prev Med* 18(3 Suppl):96–102.

Barrow GW, Saha S. 1988. Menstrual irregularity and stress fractures in collegiate female distance runners. *Am J Sports Med* 16(3):209–216.

Bell NS, Mangione TW, Hemenway D, Amoroso PJ, Jones BH. 2000. High injury rates among female army trainees: A function of gender? *Am J Prev Med* 18(3 Suppl):141–146.

Bensel CK, Kish RN. 1983. *Lower extremity disorders among men and women in Army basic training and effects of two types of boots.* Natick. TR-83/026.

Brudvig TJ, Gudger TD, Obermeyer L. 1983. Stress fractures in 295 trainees: A one-year study of incidence as related to age, sex, and race. *Mil Med* 148(8):666–667.

Brunet ME, Cook SD, Brinker MR, Dickinson JA. 1990. A survey of running injuries in 1505 competitive and recreational runners. *J Sports Med Phys Fitness* 30(3):307–315.

Canham ML, Knapik JJ, Smutok MA, Jones BH. 1998. Training, physical performance, and injuries among men and women preparing for occupations in the Army. In: Kumar S, ed. *Advances in Occupational Ergonomics and Safety: Proceedings of the XIIIth Annual International Occupational Ergonomics and Safety Conference*. Amsterdam, The Netherlands: IOS Press. Pp. 711–714.

Carlson SA, Hootman JM, Powell KE, Macera CA, Heath GW, Gilchrist J, Kimsey CD Jr, Kohl HW III. 2006. Self-reported injury and physical activity levels: United States 2000 to 2002. *Ann Epidemiol* 16(9):712–719.

Caspersen CJ, Powell KE, Christenson GM. 1985. Physical activity, exercise, and physical fitness: Definitions and distinctions for health-related research. *Public Health Reports* 100(2):126–131.

Colbert LH, Hootman JM, Macera CA. 2000. Physical activity-related injuries in walkers and runners in the aerobics center longitudinal study. *Clin J Sport Med*10(4):259–263.

Cowan DN, Robinson JR, Jones BH, Polly DW, Jr., Berrey BH. 1994. Consistency of visual assessments of arch height among clinicians. *Foot Ankle Int* 15(4):213–217.

Cowan DN, Jones BH, Frykman PN, Polly DW Jr, Harman EA, Rosenstein RM, Rosenstein MT. 1996. Lower limb morphology and risk of overuse injury among male infantry trainees. *Med Sci Sports Exerc* 28(8):945–952.

D'hondt NE, Struijs PA, Kerkhoffs GM, Verheul C, Lysens R, Aufdemkampe G, Van Dijk CN. 2002/2005. Orthotic devices for treating patellofemoral pain syndrome. *Cochrane Database Syst Rev* 2:CD002267.

Fradkin AJ, Gabbe BJ, Cameron PA. 2006. Does warming up prevent injury in sport? The evidence from randomised control trials. *J Med Sci Sport* 9(3):214–220.

Gardner LI Jr, Dziados JE, Jones BH, Brundage JF, Harris JM, Sullivan R, Gill P. 1988. Prevention of lower extremity stress fractures: A controlled trial of a shock absorbent insole. *Am J Public Health* 78(12):1563–1567.

Garrick JG, Gillien DM, Whiteside P. 1986. The epidemiology of aerobic dance injuries. *Am J Sports Med* 14(1):67–72.

Giladi M, Milgrom C, Danon Y, Aharonson Z. 1985. The correlation between cumulative march training and stress fractures in soldiers. *Mil Med* 150(11):600–601.

Herbert RD, Gabriel M. 2002. Effects of stretching before and after exercising on muscle soreness and risk of injury: Systematic review. *BMJ* 325(7362):468.

Hootman JM, Macera CA, Ainsworth BE, Martin M, Addy CL, Blair SN. 2001. Association among physical activity level, cardiorespiratory fitness, and risk of musculoskeletal injury. *Am J Epidemiol* 154(3):251–258.

Hootman JM, Macera CA, Ainsworth BE, Martin M, Addy CL, Blair SN. 2002. Predictors of lower extremity injury among recreationally active adults. *Clin J Sport Med* 12(2):99–106.

Hurley MV. 1999. The role of muscle weakness n the pathogenesis of osteoarthritis. *Rheum Dis Clin North Am* 25(2):283–298.

Jones BH, Bovee MW, Knapik JJ. 1992. Associations among body composition, physical fitness, and injury in men and women Army trainees. In: Marriott BM, Grumstrup-Scott J, eds. *Body Composition and Physical Performance: Applications for the Military Services*. Washington, DC: National Academy Press. Pp. 141–173.

Jones BH, Bovee MW, Harris JM III, Cowan DN. 1993a. Intrinsic risk factors for exercise-related injuries among male and female Army trainees. *Am J Sports Med* 21(5):705–710.

Jones BH, Cowan DN, Tomlinson JP, Robinson JR, Polly DW, Frykman PN. 1993b. Epidemiology of injuries associated with physical training among young men in the Army. *Med Sci Sports Exerc* 25(2):197–203.

Jones BH, Cowan DN, Knapik JJ. 1994. Exercise, training and injuries. *Sports Med* 18(3):202–214.

Jones BH, Thacker SB, Gilchrist J, Kimsey CD, Jr., Sosin DM. 2002. Prevention of lower extremity stress fractures in athletes and soldiers: A systematic review. *Epidemiol Rev* 24(2):228–247.

Knapik JJ, Jones BH, Bauman CL, Harris JM. 1992. Strength, flexibility and athletic injuries. *Sports Med* 14(5):277–288.

Knapik J, Ang P, Reynolds K, Jones B. 1993. Physical fitness, age, and injury incidence in infantry soldiers. *J Occup Med* 35(6):598–603.

Knapik JJ, Sharp MA, Canham ML, Hauret K, Cuthie J, Hewitson W, Hoedebecke E, Lauren MJ, Polyak C, Carroll D, Jones B. 1998. *Injury Incidence and Risk Factors Among U.S. Army Basic Trainees (Including Fitness Training Unit Personnel, Discharges, and Newstarts) at Ft. Jackson, SC, 1998.* USACHPPM Technical Report. 29-HE-8370-98. Aberdeen Proving Ground, MD: U.S. Army Center for Health Promotion and Preventive Medicine.

Knapik JJ, Sharp MA, Canham-Chervak M, Hauret K, Patton JF, Jones BH. 2001. Risk factors for training-related injuries among men and women in basic combat training. *Med Sci Sports Exerc* 33(6):946–954.

Knapik JJ, Hauret KG, Arnold S, Canham-Chervak M, Mansfield AJ, Hoedebecke EL, McMillian D. 2003. Injury and fitness outcomes during implementation of physical readiness training. *Int J Sports Med* 24(5):372–381.

Knapik JJ, Bullock SH, Canada S, Toney E, Wells JD, Hoedebecke E, Jones BH. 2004a. Influence of an injury reduction program on injury and fitness outcomes among soldiers. *Inj Prev* 10(1):37–42.

Knapik JJ, Darakjy S, Scott S, Hauret KG, Canada S, Marin R, Palkoska F, VanCamp S, Piskator E, Rieger W, Jones BH. 2004b. *Evaluation of Two Army Fitness Programs: The TRADOC Standardized Physical Training Program for Basic Combat Training and the Fitness Assessment Program.* USACHPPM Technical Report 12-HF-5772B-04. Aberdeen Proving Ground, MD: U.S. Army Center for Health Promotion and Preventive Medicine.

Knapik J, Darakjy S, Scott S, Hauret KG, Canada S, Marin R, Rieger W, Jones BH. 2005. Evaluation of a standardized physical training program for basic combat training. *J Strength Cond Res* 19(2):246–253.

Knapik JJ, Scott SJ, Sharp MA, Hauret KG, Darakjy S, Rieger WR, Palkoska FA, VanCamp SE, Jones, BH. 2006. The basis for prescribed ability group run speeds and distances in U.S. Army basic training. *Mil Med* 171(7):669–677.

Konradsen L, Hansen EB, Sondergaard L. 1990. Long-distance running and osteoarthritis. *Am J Sports Med* 18(4):379–381.

Koplan JP, Powell KE, Sikes RK, Shirley RW, Campbell CC. 1982. An epidemiologic study of the benefits and risks of running. *J Am Med Assoc* 248(23):3118–3121.

Koplan JP, Siscovick DS, Goldbaum GM. 1985. The risks of exercise: A public health view of injuries and hazards. *Public Health Reports* 100(2):189–195.

Kowal DM. 1980. Nature and causes of injuries in women resulting from an edurance training program. *Am J Sports Med* 8(4):265–269.

Lloyd T, Triantafyllou SJ, Baker ER, Houts PS, Whiteside JA, Kalenak A, Stumpf PG. 1986. Women athletes with menstrual irregularity have increased musculoskeletal injuries. *Med Sci Sports Exerc* 18(4):374–379.

Macera CA, Pate RR, Powell KE, Jackson KL, Kendrick JS, Craven TE. 1989. Predicting lower-extremity injuries among habitual runners. *Arch Intern Med* 149(11):2565–2568.

Maffulli N, King JB. 1992. Effects of physical activity on some components of the skeletal system. *Sports Med* 13(6):393–407.

Maganaris CN, Narici MV, Almekinders LC, Maffulli N. 2004. Biomechanics and pathophysiology of overuse tendon injuries: Ideas on insertional tendinopathy. *Sports Med* 34(14):1005–1017.

Marti B, Vader JP, Minder CE, Abelin T. 1988. On the epidemiology of running injuries. The 1984 Bern Grand-Prix study. *Am J Sports Med* 16(3):285–294.

McKean KA, Manson NA, Stanish WD. 2006. Musculoskeletal injury in the masters runners. *Clin J Sport Med* 16(2):149–154.

Mittleman MA, Maclure M, Tofler GH, Sherwood JB, Goldberg RJ, Muller JE. 1993. Triggering of acute myocardial infarction by heavy physical exertion: protection against triggering by regular exertion. *N Engl J Med* 329(23):1677–1683.

NRC (National Research Council). 2006. Physical fitness and musculoskeletal injury. In: Sackett PR, Mavor AS, eds. *Assessing Fitness for Military Enlistment: Physical, Medical, and Mental Health Standards.* Washington, DC: The National Academies Press. Pp. 66–108.

Parkkari J, Kannus P, Natri A, Lapinleimu I, Palvanen M, Heiskanen M, Vuori I, Jarvinen M. 2004. Active living and injury risk. *Int J Sports Med* 25(3):209–216.

Pollock ML, Gettman LR, Milesis CA, Bah MD, Durstine L, Johnson RB. 1977. Effects of frequency and duration of training on attrition and incidence of injury. *Med Sci Sports* 9(1):31–36.

Rauh MJ, Koepsell TD, Rivara FP, Margherita AJ, Rice SG. 2006a. Epidemiology of musculoskeletal injuries amoung high school cross-country runners. *Am J Epidemiol* 163(2):151-159.

Rauh MJ, Macera CA, Trone DW, Shaffer RA, Brodine SK. 2006b. Epidemiology of stress fracture and lower-extremity overuse injury in female recruits. *Med Sci Sports Exerc* 38(9):1571–1577.

Requa RK, DeAvilla LN, Garrick JG. 1993. Injuries in recreational adult fitness activities. *Am J Sports Med* 21(3):461–467.

Reynolds KL, Heckel HA, Witt CE, Martin JW, Pollard JA, Knapik JJ, Jones BH. 1994. Cigarette smoking, physical fitness, and injuries in infantry soldiers. *Am J Prev Med* 10(3):145–150.

Rome K, Handoll HH, Ashford R. 2005. Interventions for preventing and treating stress fractures and stress reactions of bone of the lower limbs in young adults. *Cochrane Database Syst Rev* 2:CD000450.

Rudzki SJ, Cunningham MJ. 1999. The effect of a modified physical training program in reducing injury and medical discharge rates in Australian Army recruits. *Mil Med* 164(9):648–652.

Shaffer RA. 1996. *Musculoskeletal Injury Project*. Presented at the 43rd Annual Meeting of the American College of Sports Medicine. Cincinnati, OH.

Shaffer RA, Brodine SK, Almeida SA, Williams KM, Ronaghy S. 1999. Use of simple measures of physical activity to predict stress fractures in young men undergoing a rigorous physical training program. *Am J Epidemiol* 149(3):236–242.

Shaffer RA, Rauh MJ, Brodine SK, Trone DW, Macera CA. 2006. Predictors of stress fracture susceptibility in young female recruits. *Am J Sports Med* 34(1):108–115.

Sharma P, Maffulli N. 2006. Biology of tendon injury: Healing, modeling and remodeling. *J Musculoskelet Neuronal Interact* 6(2):181–190.

Shrier I. 1999. Stretching before exercise does not reduce the risk of local muscle injury: A critical review of the clinical and basic science literature. *Clin J Sport Med* 9(4):221–227.

Shrier I. 2004. Muscle dysfunction versus wear and tear as a cause of exercise-related osteoarthritis: An epidemiological update. *Brit J Sports Med* 38(5):526–535.

Siscovick DS, Weiss NS, Fletcher RH, Lasky T. 1984. The incidence of primary cardiac arrest during vigorous exercise. *N Engl J Med* 311(14):874–877.

Siscovick DS. 1997. Exercise and its role in sudden cardiac death. *Cardiol Clin* 15(3):467–472.

Suter E, Marti B, Gutzwiller F. 1994. Jogging or walking—comparison of health effects. *Ann Epidemiol* 4(5):375–381.

Taunton JE, Ryan MB, Clement DB, McKenzie DC, Lloyd-Smith DR, Zumbo BD. 2003. A prospective study of running injuries: The Vancouver Sun Run "In Training" clinics. *Br J Sports Med* 37(3):239–244.

Thacker SB, Gilchrist J, Stroup DF, Kimsey CD Jr. 2004. The impact of stretching on sports injury risk: A systematic review of the literature. *Med Sci Sports Exerc* 36(3):371–378.

Thelin N, Holmberg S, Thelin A. 2006. Knee injuries account for the sports-related increased risk of knee osteoarthritis. *Scand J Med Sci Sports* 16(5):329–333.

Thompson PD. 2005. Exercise prescription and proscription for patients with coronary artery disease. *Circulation* 112(15):2354–2363.

Vuori I. 1986. The cardiovascular risks of physical activity. *Acta Med Scand Suppl* 711:205–214.

Walter SD, Hart LE, McIntosh JM, Sutton JR. 1989. The Ontario cohort study of running-related injuries. *Arch Intern Med* 149(11):2561–2564.

Westphal KA, Friedl KE, Sharp MA, Kiong N, Kramer TR, Reynolds KL, Marchitelli LJ. 1995. Health, performance, and nutritional status of U.S. Army women during basic combat training: USARIEM Technical Report T96-2. Natick, MA: U.S. Army Research Institute of Environmental Medicine.

Whang W, Manson JE, Hu FB, Chae CU, Rexrode KM, Willett WC, Stampfer MJ, Albert CM. 2006. Physical exertion, exercise, and sudden cardiac death in women. *J Am Med Assoc* 295(12):1399–1403.

White JA, Wright V, Hudson AM. 1993. Relationship between habitual physical activity and osteoarthrosis in ageing women. *Public Health* 107(6):459–470.

Wilber CA, Holland GJ, Madison RE, Loy SF. 1995. An epidemiological analysis of overuse injuries among recreational cyclists. *Int J Sports Med* 16(3):201–206.

Withnall R, Eastaugh J, Freemantle N. 2006. Do shock absorbing insoles in recruits undertaking high levels of physical activity reduce lower limb injury? A randomized controlled trial. *J R Soc Med* 99(1):32–37.

Yeung EW, Yeung SS. 2001. Interventions for preventing lower limb soft-tissue injuries in runners. *Cochrane Database Syst Rev* 3:CD001256.

5

Physical Activity and Special Considerations for Children, Adolescents, and Pregnant and Postpartum Women

A number of population groups merit special attention with regard to the relationship between physical activity and health. This chapter presents evidence of the effects of physical activity on the health of school-age children and adolescents and of pregnant and postpartum women. For convenience, the term *youth* was sometimes used by the presenters to refer to school-aged children and adolescents. The discussion section presents promising evidence relating physical activity to specific outcomes in children and adolescents, information on physical activity and skeletal growth in children and adolescents, and a brief summary of points raised during the group discussion.

PHYSICAL ACTIVITY AND CHILDREN AND ADOLESCENTS

Presenter: Robert M. Malina

This presentation included background information, evidence related to the benefits of physical activity for children and adolescents, and consideration of the amount of physical activity needed by youth.

Background

It is generally presumed that regular physical activity is essential to support the normal growth and maturation, health, and fitness of children and adolescents. Fairly recently, an expert panel was formed to review the effects of physical activity on health and behavioral outcomes in school-aged children and adolescents ages 6 to 18 years. The panel also was charged with developing a recommendation for physical activity for children and adolescents. The effects of physical activity on indicators of growth and maturation were not considered. In particular, the panelists addressed the following questions:

- What are the health, fitness, and behavioral benefits of regular physical activity for school-aged children and adolescents?
- In terms of frequency, intensity, and time (duration), what amount and type of activity is needed to bring about beneficial effects on the selected indicators?
- What amount of physical activity should be recommended?

The indicators considered included measures of health, fitness, behavior, and injury risk. Panelists used a standardized evaluation format to examine the evidence. The panel report is published in *the Journal of Pediatrics* (Strong et al., 2005).

Evidence of Specific Outcomes

Adiposity

Normal weight youth Enhanced physical activity programs appear to have a minimal effect on adiposity among youth of normal weight. Cross-sectional and longitudinal comparisons of active and less active youth give equivocal results regarding skinfold measurements. Two experimental studies suggest that youth need a considerable amount of physical activity to maintain a healthy weight.

Obese youth Experimental studies of obese youth indicate a reduction in total body and visceral adiposity with regular activity. In this case, regular activity is defined as a variety of moderate to vigorous activity for 30 to 40 minutes per day on 3 to 5 days per week.

Lipids and Lipoproteins

In a variety of intervention studies of youth, weak beneficial effects of physical activity are reported for reducing the level of high-density lipoprotein cholesterol and triglycerides. The amount of physical activity needed to achieve beneficial effects appears to be a minimum of 40 minutes per day of moderate to vigorous activity for 5 days per week over a 4-month period. A sustained volume of physical activity may be a key factor. School-based programs generally were not effective in improving the lipid and lipoprotein profiles of youth.

Blood Pressure

Normotensive youth No clear association was found between physical activity and blood pressure in normotensive youth.

Hypertensive youth Experimental aerobic training programs have demonstrated beneficial effects on the blood pressure of hypertensive youth. Thirty-minute sessions of sufficient intensity to improve aerobic fitness on 3 days per week for 12 to 32 weeks provided benefit. Two studies showed no change in blood pressure with resistance training. Among youth with mild essential hypertension, some evidence suggests that aerobic programs may reduce blood pressure.

Other Indicators of Cardiovascular Health

In general, the data that physical activity may improve other indicators of cardiovascular health among youth are very limited. However, data suggest that aerobic training increases resting vagal tone as reflected in higher heart rate variability, which is a marker of cardiac parasympathetic activity. The implications of this change for the development of cardiovascular disease are uncertain.

Metabolic Syndrome and Type 2 Diabetes

Two studies indicate that insulin and triglyceride concentrations and adiposity are favorably influenced by physical activity in obese youth.

The physical activity level was moderate to vigorous three times per week. Essentially no useful data are available regarding associations of physical activity and type 2 diabetes in children and adolescents.

Skeletal Health

Evidence from a variety of studies suggests a beneficial effect of regular physical activity on bone mineral content and bone mineral density. Most of the studies have been conducted on prepubertal children or adolescents in the early stages of puberty. Typically, the studies involve moderate- to high-strain physical activity for 10 to 60 minutes per day at least 2 to 3 times per week. Some have used 10 minutes of impact activity and 45 to 60 minutes of general weight-bearing activity. Limited evidence suggests little or no positive effect after puberty.

Aerobic Fitness

In both cross-sectional and longitudinal studies, data suggest higher aerobic fitness in active youth than in less active youth. In experimental studies of children ages 8 years and older, the evidence consistently shows a favorable effect of physical activity on aerobic fitness—namely, about a 10 percent increase in peak VO_2. The programs that produced benefits involved continuous vigorous aerobic activity of various types for 30 to 45 minutes per day at least 3 days per week.

Muscular Strength and Endurance

Although the cross-sectional and longitudinal data are equivocal regarding the association of physical activity with muscular strength and endurance among youth, experimental data show significant gains with weight training 2 to 3 days per week with a rest day between sessions. The key appears to be a variety of progressive resistance activities, adult supervision, and the involvement of both reciprocal and large muscle groups.

Behavioral Outcomes

Examining evidence relating physical activity to behavioral outcomes poses a number of challenges, including a large number of outcome measures, problems with sampling, quasi-experimental studies, and various modes and combinations of activity. Physical activity is fairly strongly associated both with global self-esteem and physical self-concept. Aerobic activity generally has a small positive effect on symptoms of depression and anxiety, but the addition of cognitive behavioral modification produces a stronger positive effect.

The data on effects of physical activity on academic performance are limited, with very mixed results that tend toward the positive. Notably, quasi-experimental data indicate that the allocation of more curricular time to physical education or activity programs did not negatively influence academic achievement—even when less time was allocated to other subjects.

Risk of Injury

As discussed earlier by Drs. Jones and Hootman (see Chapter 4), physical activity increases the risk of injury. Data are limited, however, regarding associations of school, recreational, and free-time activities with injury. Comparability among studies is limited because of the challenges of accurate surveillance and reporting, the definition of injury, and exposure statistics, among other reasons.

Evidence from six studies of physical education indicates very low risk of injury in programs involving moderate to vigorous activity for 10 to 40 minutes on 3 days per week. In a study of self-reported injuries in recreational and sporting activities among Australian adolescents, about one in four students reported an injury, and the rate of injury was one per three instances of participation (Grimmer et al., 2000). Most (72 percent) of the injuries were classified as minor (e.g., bruises, aches, strains) and 5 percent as major (e.g., fracture, dislocation, concussion).

Summary of the Evidence on Physical Activity and Youth

The expert panel that addressed the benefits of physical activity in children and adolescents (Strong et al., 2005) determined that dose–

response data are limited. The evidence base is strongest for skeletal health, aerobic fitness, muscular strength and endurance, adiposity in the obese, and blood pressure in the hypertensive. Evidence is suggestive for adiposity and lipids in nonobese youth; for blood pressure in normotensive youth; and for self-concept, anxiety and depression symptoms, and academic performance. Data on associations of physical activity with metabolic syndrome, type 2 diabetes, and some indicators of cardiovascular health currently are very limited for youth.

Most of the experimental intervention protocols used a continuous activity program, but the activities of children, especially young children, are primarily intermittent. Figure 5-1 illustrates how activity needs vary with age during childhood and adolescence. This suggests the need to develop activity protocols that examine the effects of high-intensity, intermittent activity on indicators of health, fitness, and behaviors.

A difficulty in evaluating the effects of activity on indicators of health and fitness in children and adolescents relates to the fact that the outcome variables change with normal growth, maturation, and development, whether or not the individual is physically active on a regular basis (Malina et al., 2004; Malina and Katzmarzyk, 2006). Available data do not consider interindividual differences in maturity status and progress, especially during the adolescent years. Data also are needed on the persistence of activity-induced beneficial effects and on the amount of activity needed to maintain these beneficial effects.

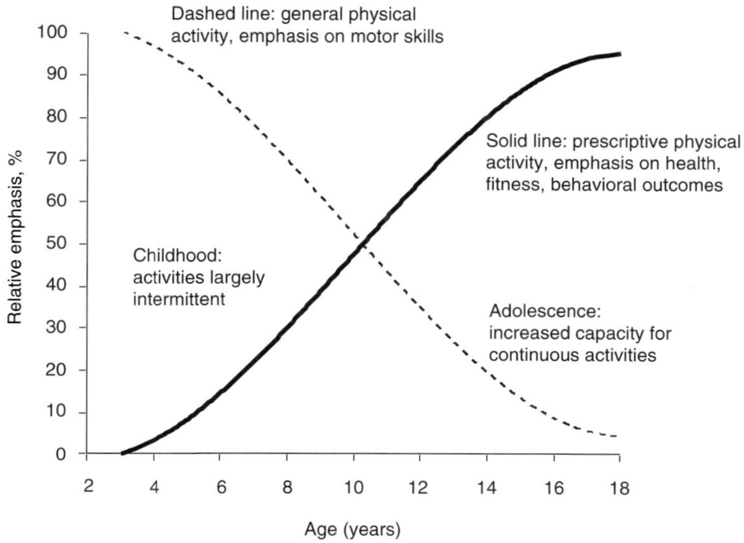

FIGURE 5-1 Changes in types of activity needs with increasing age of children and youth.
SOURCE: From R.M. Malina, 1991, Fitness and Performance: Adult Health and the Culture of Youth. In *New Possibilities, New Paradigms? American Academy of Physical Education No. 24,* edited by R.J. Park and H. M. Eckert, pages 30-38. © 1991 by American Academy of Physical Education. Adapted with permission from the American Academy of Kinesiology and Physical Education and Human Kinetics (Champaign, IL).

Concluding Remarks

In closing, Dr. Malina highlighted the importance of investigating how to prevent unhealthy weight gain in children and adolescents, considering physical inactivity as well as physical activity. Inactivity and activity have different meanings and contexts in children and youth, and they are generally independent of each other.

PHYSICAL ACTIVITY DURING PREGNANCY AND THE POSTPARTUM PERIOD

Presenter: James M. Pivarnik

This presentation addressed the historical concern with potential harm from maternal physical activity, short-term benefits from maternal physical activity for the mother and fetus, and the role of maternal physical activity on chronic disease risk of the mother later in life.

Historical Concerns and Guidelines

Early studies on physical activity and pregnancy were concerned with harm rather than benefit. Most studies used animal models. Human studies examined cardiorespiratory responses and thermoregulation in the mother, heart rate of the fetus, and outcomes of pregnancy such as birth weight, gestational length, and adverse events.

The American College of Obstetricians and Gynecologists (ACOG) developed the first exercise guidelines for pregnant women in 1985 (ACOG, 1985). Those guidelines were based on the early studies and were conservative. They included a maximum heart rate of 140 beats per minute and time limits for physical activity. The potential need for individualization of the recommendations was noted.

Between 1985 and 1994, nearly 600 relevant studies were published, most of which focused mainly on doing no harm. Many of these were laboratory studies with small sample sizes, and most involved acute maternal responses to exercise. The data suggested (1) no detrimental effects of the exercise to the mother or fetus, (2) possible reduced length of labor, (3) possible improvement in gestational diabetes mellitus (GDM), and (4) relatively little loss of fitness by chronic exercisers. The use of a target heart rate was found to be somewhat problematic because of inconsistent influences of pregnancy on heart rate among women. ACOG updated its guidance for exercise during pregnancy in 1994 (ACOG, 1994) and again 8 years later (ACOG, 2002).

Current Evidence Relating Physical Activity to Outcomes

More recently, a number of studies have examined whether maternal physical activity affects birth weight. Perkins and colleagues (2005) performed a meta-analysis of the effect of maternal physical activity on birth weight, stratified by exercise intensity. They found a slightly lighter (but not low) mean birth weight for infants born to women who took part in vigorous activity (see Figure 5-2). The topic merits attention because in the year 2000 more than two-thirds of women in the childbearing years took part in some type of physical activity (Evenson, 2004), and many women want to continue these activities during pregnancy.

Information on vigorous activity during pregnancy is very limited. In 2005, an expert panel was assembled to examine the impact of physical activity during pregnancy and the postpartum period on chronic disease risk (Pivarnik et al., 2006). That panel addressed a number of topics, including the association of physical activity with the risk of preeclampsia and with the risk of GDM. Regular physical activity in early pregnancy is associated with a reduced risk of preeclampsia in two case–control studies (Marcoux et al., 1989; Sorenson et al., 2003) and one cohort study (Saftlas et al., 2004). The evidence is not strong, but it is in the same direction. Although pilot data from Mottola and colleagues (2005) show a slightly reduced rate of GDM in overweight pregnant women who began a program of physical activity, data are insufficient to develop specific optimal physical activity guidelines for GDM prevention.

Some evidence is available regarding the role of physical activity in postpartum weight reduction. Larson-Meyer (2002) reviewed approximately 60 cross-sectional and randomized trials on this topic, looking at postpartum exercise but not activity performed during pregnancy. When compared to sedentary women, those who performed moderate physical activity without caloric restriction did not appear to show greater weight or fat loss. In a later report, Rooney et al. (2005) evaluated nearly 800 women early in pregnancy and followed them for 15 years. Disease and risk factor development (i.e., diabetes, heart disease, dyslipidemia, and hypertension) were positively related to weight gain over the 15 years. The women who continued to perform aerobic exercise postpartum were less likely to become obese than those who did not. Among factors that can create barriers to postpartum physical activity are lack of time and lack of child care (Beilock et al., 2001).

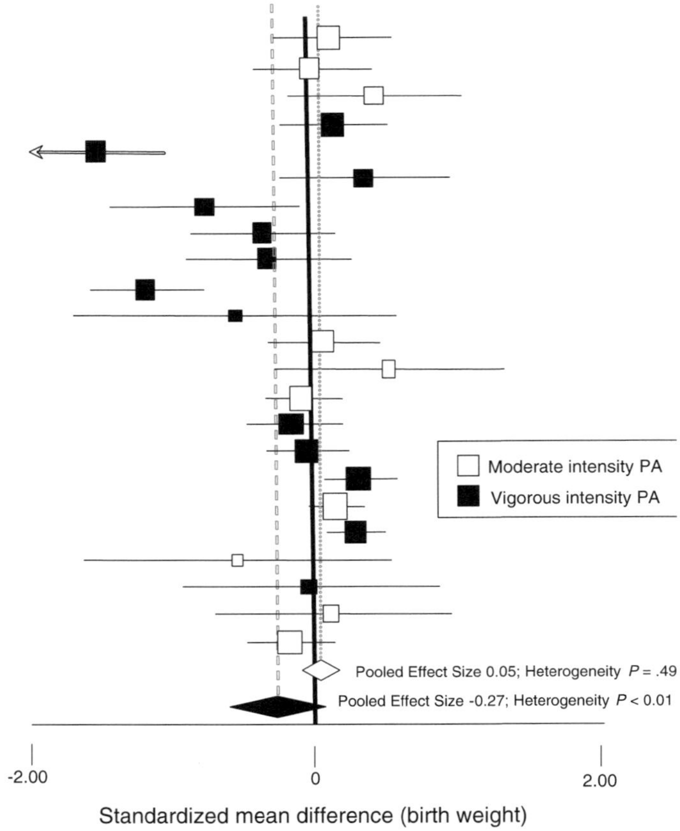

FIGURE 5-2 Effect of maternal physical activity on birth weight, stratified by exercise intensity. The sizes of the boxes reflect the relative sample sizes.
NOTE: PA = physical activity. The studies represented by the boxes in the figure are listed in descending order as follows: Beckmann and Beckmann, 1990; Bell et al., 1995; Botkin and Driscoll, 1991; Clapp, 1990, 1996; Clapp and Dickstein, 1984; Clapp et al., 1998, 1999, 2000; Collings et al., 1983; Homs et al., 1996; Lewis et al., 1998; Magann et al., 1996, 2002; Marquez-Sterling et al., 2000; Pivarnik et al., 1994; Rice and Fort, 1991; Stemfeld, 1997.
SOURCE: Perkins et al. (2005).

Concluding Remarks

Dr. Pivarnik identified the effects of maternal recreational exercise on the health, growth, and development of the offspring as an exciting new topic of research. Dr. Jim Clapp is a lead investigator in this area, but few studies are available and sample sizes are small. Initial studies indicate that beginning or continuing recreational exercise during pregnancy has no identifiable acute or chronic adverse effects on the offspring and may have some positive effects. There is a great need for prospective, randomized exercise-intervention studies in diverse populations.

DISCUSSION

Promising Lines of Evidence Relating Physical Activity to Outcomes in Children and Youth

Discussant: Russell R. Pate

There is much less evidence supporting the development of physical activity guidelines for children and youth than there is for adults. The young age group poses enormous research design challenges for two major reasons: (1) most young persons are healthy and remain so during childhood and adolescence, and (2) young people are the most active segment of our society. These two factors make it very difficult to demonstrate positive health effects. In view of these factors and the data presented by Dr. Malina, Dr. Pate suggested directing attention to the following three topics:

1. *The amount of activity sustained over time that minimizes the risk of excessive weight gain over that period.* This focus could be valuable in part because the increased prevalence of obesity is of concern to society at large. A few U.S. studies and more European studies have addressed activity and weight gain over time in children and youth of normal weight.
2. *Activity related to fitness.* Children and youth with low fitness levels tend to have low fitness during adulthood, and evidence shows a strong association of low adult fitness with a range of chronic disease outcomes (see Chapter 2). Using data from the

National Health and Nutrition Examination Survey, Dr. Pate's group recently found that about one-third of U.S. children and youth fail to meet aerobic fitness standards. Moreover, Dr. Malina reported that the literature on this topic is fairly extensive.

3. *Activity and the multiple metabolic syndrome*. This is a rapidly developing area, and it is possible that evidence will be available soon regarding protective levels of physical activity.

Physical Activity and the Skeleton in Children and Youth

Discussant: Heather McKay

Topics addressed in this discussion include the optimal period for a response of bone to exercise, bone geometry related to bone strength, modes and intensity of exercise, and the benefits of muscular strength for the skeleton.

Timing

Childhood is an essential time to introduce physical activity in terms of healthy growth of the skeleton. The key time appears to be early puberty. Bone mineral content velocity lags behind peak growth and peak linear growth by about 8 months. Approximately 26 percent of one's adult skeleton is accrued in the 2 years around the age of peak skeletal growth (age 11.8 years for girls and 13.4 years for boys). This amount of accrual represents as much bone as most people will lose in their entire adult lives (Arlot et al., 1997).

Mechanical Loading and Bone Geometry

Stress causes strain on bones. Bone is accrued primarily on the periosteal (outer) surface, meaning that the bone is getting larger (Turner and Robling, 2003). An increase of as little as one millimeter in the outer surface of bone increases strength substantially. Bone may alter its geometric properties independently of changes in bone mass (Jarvinen et al., 1999). Adding bone to the outside increases strength, and adding bone to the endosteal (inner) surface increases strength also. Dual-energy X-ray absorptiometry (DEXA) does not detect these responses. Bone mineral density by DEXA may be the same across different configurations of a cross section of bone, even though strengths may differ by four or eight times. Thus there is a huge gap between knowing the amount of bone mineral in a given bone and knowing its structural capacity. The whole bone structure substantiates the mechanical competence of bone (Jarvinen et al., 2005).

Modes and Intensity of Exercise

Data are lacking on what mode or intensity of physical activity is osteogenic (builds bone). Studies with rats indicate that 5 jumps per day were as effective as 40 jumps per day in increasing bone strength (Umemura et al., 1997). Preliminary data from Dr. McKay's group suggest that taking five jumps each of three times per day during school increases distal tibia muscular strength in boys but not in girls.

Muscular Strength and the Skeleton

In both males and females, peak lean mass accrual occurs about 4 to 6 months before peak bone mass accrual (Rauch et al., 2004). Data show a very close relationship between a surrogate for muscle strength, total lean body mass, and bone strength. Similarly there is a close association between an increase in muscle mass and an increase in bone mass. Thus interventions that increase muscular strength also may benefit the skeleton.

Concluding Remarks

Dr. McKay highlighted the following points:

- Early puberty is the period when the response of bone to exercise is optimized.
- Small changes in bone geometry result in substantial increases in bone strength.

- Frequent episodes of short exercise bouts may be as effective as sustained exercise.
- Further studies are needed.
- Schools may be the key avenue to having an impact on children's health.
- The benefits of exercise do not persist if exercise is withdrawn.

GROUP DISCUSSION

Moderator: Patty S. Freedson

Among the points raised during discussion were the following:

- The quantification of intermittent bouts of physical activity may pose a challenge. Accelerometry may be helpful, as may other new technological approaches to assess behavior objectively.
- Questions were raised about the appropriateness of an exercise prescription model for children. Considering a diversity of activities may be helpful, along with setting appropriate targets for the duration of moderate to vigorous intensity activity.
- More data are needed about the risk of physical activity among children and youth.
- Work in animals suggests that dividing loads over several sessions per day substantially increases the osteogenic response. Evidence regarding this relationship in humans is needed.

REFERENCES

ACOG (American College of Obstetricians and Gynecologists). 1985. *Technical Bulletin: Exercise During Pregnancy and the Postnatal Period*. Washington, DC: ACOG.

ACOG. 1994. *Technical Bulletin No. 173, Women and Exercise*. Washington, DC: ACOG.

ACOG. 2002. Exercise during pregnancy and the postpartum period. ACOG Committee Opinion 267. *Obstet Gynecol* 99(1):171–173.

Arlot ME, Sornay-Rendu E, Garnero P, Vey-Marty B, Delmas PD. 1997. Apparent pre- and postmenopausal bone loss evaluated by DXA at different skeletal sites in women: The OFELY cohort. *J Bone Miner Res* 12(4): 683–690.

Beilock, SL, Feltz DL, Pivarnik JM. 2001. Training patterns of athletes during pregnancy and postpartum. *Res Q Exerc Sport* 72(1):39–46.

Evenson KR, Savitz DA, Huston SL. 2004. Leisure-time physical activity among pregnant women in the US. *Paediatr Perinat Epidemiol* 18(6): 400–407.

Grimmer KA, Jones D, Williams J. 2000. Prevalence of adolescent injury from recreational exercise: An Australian perspective. *Adolesc Health* 27(4): 266–272.

Jarvinen TL, Kannus P, Sievanen H. 1999. Have the DXA-based exercise studies seriously underestimated the effects of mechanical loading on bone? *J Bone Miner Res* 14(9):634–1635.

Jarvinen TL, Sievanen H, Jokihaara J, Einhorn TA. 2005. Revival of bone strength: The bottom line. *J Bone Miner Res* 20(5):717–720.

Larson-Meyer DE. 2002. Effect of postpartum exercise on mothers and their offspring: A review of the literature. *Obes Res* 10(8):841–853.

Malina RM. 1991. Fitness and performance: Adult health and the culture of youth. In: Park RJ, Eckert HM. Eds. *New Possibilities, New Paradigms?* American Academy of Physical Education Papers No. 24. Champaign, IL: Human Kinetics. Pp. 30–38.

Malina RM, Bouchard C, Bar-Or O. 2004. *Growth, Maturation, and Physical Activity*, 2nd edition. Champaign, IL: Human Kinetics.

Malina RM, Katzmarzyk PT. 2006. Physical activity and fitness in an international growth standard for preadolescent and adolescent children. *Food and Nutrition Bulletin* 27(Suppl 4):S295–S313.

Marcoux S, Brisson J, Fabia J. 1989. The effect of leisure time physical activity on the risk of preeclampsia and gestational hypertension. *J Epidemiol Community Health* 43:147–152.

Mottola MF, Sopper MM, Vanderspank D, Charlesworth S, Hanley A. 2005. Insulin sensitivity is maintained in late pregnancy among overweight women at risk for gestational diabetes participating in a Nutrition and Exercise Lifestyle Intervention Program (NELIP). *Can Federation Biological Societies Proceedings*. Pp. 62.

Perkins CD, Pivarnik JM, Reeves MJ, Feltz DL, Womack CJ. 2005. Maternal physical activity and birth-weight: A meta-analysis. *Med Sci Sports Exerc* 37(Suppl 5):S177.

Pivarnik JM, Chambliss HO, Clapp JF, Dugan SA, Hatch MC, Lovelady CA, Mottola MF, Williams MA. 2006. Impact of physical activity during pregnancy and postpartum on chronic disease risk. *Med Sci Sports Exerc* 38(5):989–1006.

Rauch F, Bailey DA, Baxter-Jones A, Mirwald R, Faulkner R. 2004. The 'muscle-bone unit' during the pubertal growth spurt. *Bone* 34(5):771–775.

Rooney BL, Schauberger CW, Mathiason MA. 2005. Impact of perinatal weight change on long-term obesity and obesity-related illnesses. *Obstet Gynecol* 106(6):1349–1356.

Saftlas AF, Logsden-Sackett N, Wang W, Woolson R, Bracken MB. 2004. Work, leisure-time physical activity, and risk of preeclampsia and gestational hypertension. *Am J Epidemiol* 160(8):758–765.

Sorensen TK, Williams MA, Lee I-M, Dashow EE, Thompson ML, Luthy DA. 2003. Recreational physical activity during pregnancy and risk of preeclampsia. *Hypertension* 41(6):1273–1280.

Strong WB, Malina RM, Blimkie CJR, Daniels SR, Dishman RK, Gutin B, Hergenroeder AC, Must A, Nixon PA, Pivarnik JM, Rowland T, Trost S, Trudeau F. 2005. Evidence-based physical activity for school-age youth. *J Pediatr* 146(6):732–737.

Turner CH, Robling AG. 2003. Designing exercise regimens to increase bone strength. *Exerc Sport Sci Rev* 31(1):45–50.

Umemura Y, Ishiko T, Yamauchi T, Kurono M, Mashiko S. 1997. Five jumps per day increase bone mass and breaking force in rats. *J Bone Miner Res* 12(9):1480–1485.

6

Physical Activity and Special Considerations for Older Adults

This chapter addresses the aging U.S. population, physiological changes that older people experience as they age, evidence of the benefits from physical activity, and the rationale for developing more specific physical activity guidelines targeted toward older Americans. Specific evidence was presented detailing the role of physical activity in the development of age-associated impairments, functional limitations, physical disability, and cognitive decline.

PHYSICAL ACTIVITY AND OLDER ADULTS

Presenter: Roger A. Fielding[1]

This presentation provided background information on demographic changes in the U.S. population and the prevalence of physical *inactivity* in the elderly. Then Dr. Fielding covered age-related changes in physiological function, available evidence for benefits of physical activity, research needs, and reasons to develop specific physical activity guidelines for older Americans.

[1]Dr. Fielding acknowledged support from U.S. Department of Agriculture 54-K01-01, National Institute of Aging (NIA) AG 18844, NIA AG 25270, and NIA AG 22376.

Background

The U.S. population is aging, with a projected sharp increase in the number of people over age 65 years. The rate of growth in the size of the group that is older than 85 years is even faster than that for persons over age 65 years. The over-85 age group is the fastest growing segment of our population. The prevalence of physical inactivity is highest among the elderly. Data from the Centers for Disease Control and Prevention (CDC, 2005) indicate that close to 40 percent of persons age 70 years or older have no physical activity beyond daily functioning. Similarly, Manson et al. (2004) found that more than 60 percent of persons older than 75 reported no leisure-time physical activity.

Age-Related Changes in Physiological Function

The disablement pathway originally described by Nagi (1965) and later adapted by Verbrugge and Jette (1994) includes the following steps:

1. Pathology (e.g., type II muscle fiber atrophy) →
2. Impairment (e.g., loss of muscle strength) →
3. Functional limitation (e.g., loss of mobility) →
4. Disability in which the person has a limitation in performing a socially defined role within the social or physical environment.

This model has been useful in compartmentalizing the potential effects of physical activity on age-associated functional limitations and disability. Evidence suggests that physical activity by older persons may lead to improvements at the levels of functional limitations and disability by mechanistically improving physiological function at the pathology or impairment level. Functional limitations generally are assessed either by self-report or performance-based measures, while disability usually is assessed with self-reported instruments.

Sarcopenia

Decline in skeletal muscle mass (sarcopenia) is an obvious change that occurs with aging. Scanning a cross-sectional area of the mid-thigh by computed tomography (CT) or magnetic resonance imaging (MRI) reveals that even non-obese older women have a smaller amount of muscle and more fat than do younger women. The New Mexico Elder Health Survey used dual energy X-ray absoptiometry (DEXA) scans to estimate the prevalence of sarcopenia. Selected data showing the range for men and women appear in Table 6-1. In that survey, sarcopenia was defined as having a DEXA value two standard deviations below normal for young individuals.

Decline in voluntary muscle strength occurs along with the decline in skeletal muscle mass and power. Metter et al. (1997) reported that upper extremity strength of persons age 85 and older was about 60 percent that of the 20-year-old group, and upper extremity power was only 40 percent that of the young group. Both strength and power are predictors of function in the elderly; however evidence is accumulating that power may be the stronger predictor of functional limitations and disability. Jette et al. (1981) showed that approximately 20 percent of men and 60 percent of women ages 75–84 years were unable to lift a 4.5 kg (10 lb) weight, which is comparable to the weight of a bag of groceries.

Evidence indicates that qualitative changes also occur in muscle. For example, the specific force of single skeletal muscle fibers—both the slow type I fibers and the fast oxidative type IIA fibers—was significantly lower for older men than for younger men (Frontera et al., 2000).

Aerobic Capacity

Data from a number of studies suggest that aerobic capacity declines about 1 percent per year after the third decade (Astrand, 1960; Fleg et al. 2005). Recent evidence from Fleg and colleagues (2005) suggests that longitudinal declines in aerobic capacity are independent of participation in regular physical activity and that declines in aerobic capacity in late life may be even more precipitous. The change is closely related to the age-associated decline in maximal cardiac output and parallels the

TABLE 6-1 Range of Prevalence[a] of Sarcopenia for Older Non-Hispanic White Men and Women

	---Percent---	
Age group, years	Males (n=205)	Females (n=173)
70–74	20	33
> 80	53	43

[a]Prevalence assessed by dual-energy X-ray absorptiometry in the New Mexico Elder Health Survey.
SOURCE: Adapted from Baumgartner et al. (1998).

decline in skeletal muscle oxidative capacity, as measured by decreased mitochondrial number and function. Because of these declines, even normal activities of daily living may require near maximal effort for many older people. Despite the fact that aerobic capacity does seem to decline with age, older adults who are aerobically fit have maximal capacity for oxygen consumption (VO_2max) similar to that of sedentary younger adults.

Evidence of Benefits of Physical Activity

Many studies have shown that exercise can have beneficial effects by reducing the risk of chronic diseases and mitigating signs and symptoms of disease that are already present in older adults.

Strength and Muscle Mass

A randomized controlled trial of strength training showed a progressive significant increase in muscle strength in the resistance training group throughout the year of the study, and a slight, nonsignificant increase in the control group (see Figure 6-1) (Nelson et al., 1994). Muscle mass also increased in the resistance training group.

A randomized controlled trial of nursing home residents with a mean age of 85 years found that the group that received exercise alone became stronger than the control group, but there was no improvement in muscle mass (Fiatarone et al., 1994). In contrast, the group that received exercise plus a nutritional supplement benefited in both strength and muscle mass.

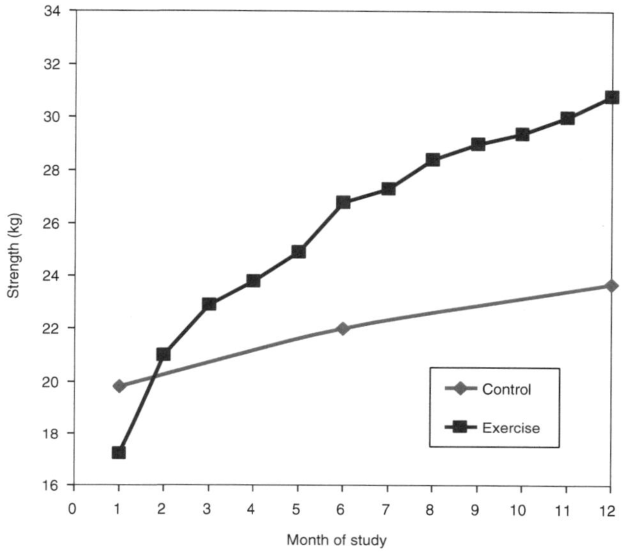

FIGURE 6-1 Effect of resistance training (lateral pull down) on muscle strength over time, postmenopausal women ages 50–70 years.
SOURCE: Morganti et al. (1995). Reprinted, with permission, from *Med Sci Sports Exerc.*

Functional Limitations and Disability

In a systematic review of effects of progressive resistance training interventions, Latham et al. (2004) reported on changes in functional limitations and disability among older individuals who were impaired at baseline. In the pooled analysis, improvements in strength were moderate to large, and improvements in functional limitations (gait speed, chair stand, and 6-minute walk) were modest to moderate. No effect of resistance training was seen, however, in a physical function subscale or in the measure of activities of daily living. The changes in functional limitations were variable and may depend on baseline performance, stimulus intensity, and duration.

In a recently released report on the Lifestyle Interventions and Independence for Elders Pilot (LIFE-P) study (a 1-year program of combined aerobic, strength, and balance training in older men and women with functional limitations at baseline) showed significant and clinically meaningful improvements in the short physical performance battery score compared to a health education control group (The LIFE Investigators, 2006).

Another systematic review of the impact of resistance training on the disablement process (Keysor and Jette, 2001) found that 23 of the 26 studies demonstrated improved strength, and over half showed improvement in functional tasks such as walking and stair climbing. Only a few studies, however, showed improvement in physical disability, and those improvements were small to modest.

Limitations in instruments designed to measure disability may explain, at least in part, why most physical activity studies fail to show an impact on disability. Using a newly developed instrument to assess disability in intervention studies, Dr. Fielding's group conducted a 12-week randomized trial of the effect of progressive resistance training on disability in older persons who had experienced a stroke. Strength increased about 16 to 38 percent in the exercise group compared to no change in the attention control group. In addition, data collected using the Late Life Function and Disability Instrument, which was developed and validated by Jette et al. (2002), showed improvements to the advanced lower extremity function domain and two domains of disability (limitation and instrumental role) (Ouellette, 2004).

Falls

Falls are a precipitating event for fracture. Approximately 50 to 65 percent of all falls occur in or around the home (Cummings et al., 1995). Most occur on the same level, from a standing height, as by tripping while walking rather than falling down stairs. Some evidence indicates that physical activity or a combination of balance and strengthening activity programs may reduce falls in older individuals. For example, in a randomized trial involving frail older women, Campbell et al. (1997) found that 30 minutes of home-based strength and balance exercises three times per week over 1 year resulted in significant improvements over the control group in chair stand time (the time to stand up from a standard chair five times) and balance measures. In addition, the exercise group had a significant 40 percent decrease in injurious falls.

Cognitive Function

In a review, Kramer et al. (2006) reported that observational studies suggest an association between physical activity in persons with normal cognitive decline and the development of Alzheimer's disease and other dementias. However, the studies generally covered a short period of evaluation (2 to 8 years). Intervention studies suggest that exercise training has a positive effect on executive control processes. These processes include planning, scheduling, working memory, and multitasking.

Mean differences in baseline cognitive function scores showed a significant value for trend by quartile of walking for four of five tests of cognitive function (Weuve et al., 2004). Two meta-analyses have been conducted of intervention trials that address physical activity and cognitive function (Colcombe and Kramer, 2003; Heyn et al., 2004). In non-demented older adults, the estimated effect size was 0.48; and in demented elderly patients, the effect size was similar (0.57). Dr. Fielding highlighted the need to conduct more basic studies to identify the areas of the brain that are activated by exercise and the mechanisms of action by which exercise exerts its effects.

Concluding Remarks

In closing, Dr. Fielding provided his perspective on information needs and on reasons for specific physical activity guidelines for older Americans.

Research Needs

Among the research needs relating to physical activity in older adults are the following:

- A definitive randomized trial of physical activity on disability outcomes
- Evidence of the ability of older individuals with functional limitations to adhere to physical activity recommendations
- Better understanding of appropriate physical activities to improve balance
- Definitive studies on exercise and cognition

Rationale for Developing Specific Physical Activity Guidelines for Older Americans

Specificity is needed to address the unique changes in physiological reserve that occur with aging. This is especially important if guidelines will be developed to apply to older individuals with several comorbidities and functional limitations, as well as to older healthy persons. Older persons have more medical conditions and comorbidities than do younger persons, and they are at increased risk of injury. In addition, long-term adherence to physical participation can be an issue, especially for older adults with functional limitations. In the LIFE-P study (The LIFE Investigators, 2006), over the course of 1 year, about half the subjects had to suspend participation in moderate physical activity for a period because of a health problem. Thus effective strategies that can help older adults resume physical activity following these common health transitions merit consideration when developing physical activity guidelines for this population.

DISCUSSION

Physical Activity Guidelines for Older Adults

Discussant: Anne B. Newman

Background

In contrast with common perception, the rates of disability for activities of daily living (defined as difficulty with self-care) are rather low (about 1 to 2 percent) in older persons. Rates of loss of mobility, however, are much higher. After age 70, the rate of incident mobility *difficulty* is 10 percent per year, and about one-third of the affected individuals have severe mobility *disability* (Penninx et al., 2004). Challenges to one's ability to remain physically active with older age include risk of hip fracture, pneumonia, and congestive heart failure. The acute declines and limited recovery from such intermittent health events may further accelerate functional decline and ultimately lead to disability.

As mentioned earlier in this session by Dr. Fielding, longitudinal data show a decline in maximal oxygen consumption with aging. Although those who are active maintain higher oxygen consumption, the rate of the decline is not prevented by physical activity (Fleg et al., 2005; Metter et al., 1999). Metter et al. (1999) observed age-associated decreases in leg isometric strength and muscle mass, and Goodpaster et al. (2006) showed that loss of strength is proportionately much greater than loss of muscle mass in men and women ages 70 to 79 years.

Reasons for Developing Guidelines for Older Adults

Dr. Newman agreed with Dr. Fielding on the need for developing physical activity guidelines for older adults and highlighted the following reasons:

- Older adults are at risk for or may have multiple chronic conditions. Thus physical activity may interfere with or retard both disease pathways and age-related decline in the pathway to disability.
- Old age is a heterogeneous period of development, during which the dynamics of weight change need to be considered. Weight tends to fluctuate and decline after about age 70 years (Roberts and Williamson, 2002). Many older persons will lose weight at a low level of food intake and a very low level of energy expenditure (Newman et al., 2005).
- Older adults may not know what they can do or should do for physical activity. In the Dynamics of Health, Aging and Body Composition Study (Health ABC), only three-quarters of older adults who reported no difficulty walking a quarter of a mile could actually do so at examination (Newman et al., 2006) There is a need for a message about goals that address ability and capacity.

Need for a Consistent Message

Dr. Newman highlighted the importance of developing a consistent message that addresses the type of activity to choose for a particular benefit:

- Aerobic and/or strength training for function
- Weight-bearing and strength training activities for bone health

- Neurologically stimulating activities for balance and speeded tasks

Potentially beneficial activities not mentioned earlier include t'ai chi (Wolf et al., 1996) and dance (Verghese, 2006).

There is a need for a message about goals that address ability and for methods to measure ability. A majority of adults older than 70 years have difficulty with treadmill testing, and many cannot provide a useful self-report of their ability to walk a distance (Sayers et al., 2004). Notably, Newman et al. (2006) showed that rates of disability are inversely related to the ability to walk one-quarter mile.

Concluding Remarks

In closing, Dr. Newman underscored that older adults do benefit from physical activity. Comprehensive messages need to be developed, and the recommendations need to be individualized to the developmental period in the life course. Finally, objective assessment of the functional capacity of older adults needs to be incorporated into clinical practice for appropriate goal setting.

Group Discussion

Moderator: Miriam Nelson

Among the points raised during the discussion were the following:

- The rate of loss of aerobic capacity with age may be accelerated in older age groups. In the Baltimore Longitudinal Study of Aging, the rate of loss for persons in their seventies and eighties was approximately 20 to 30 percent per decade. Since the rate of loss is about the same for persons at different levels of fitness, it becomes even more important for inactive persons to increase their level of aerobic capacity through physical activity. Focusing efforts on prevention could help raise fitness levels above the threshold for disability, thus helping prevent disability.
- Evidence suggests that physical activity of moderate intensity may have quite robust health effects for older adults. A fair

amount of evidence from randomized controlled trials indicates health benefits at levels of physical activity that are lower than currently recommended.

- Physical activity programs for older persons can be safe and effective in community settings.
- Clinically meaningful outcome measurements are needed to assess the effectiveness of physical activity interventions in the field.
- Large randomized controlled trials are needed to determine the extent to which physical activity can reduce disability over the long term. Observational studies have serious limitations.
- The examination of adiposity—in addition to muscle mass and quality—is important in investigations of physical activity and functional limitations in disability. Carrying excess weight is an independent factor in predicting disability.
- The International Consensus Conference on Dose–Response covered a large percentage of persons older than 65 years and reported a well-documented dose–response effect. In particular, greater amounts of physical activity reduced mortality rates.

REFERENCES

Astrand I. 1960. Aerobic work capacity in men and women with special reference to age. *J Appl Physiol* 49(169):1–92.

Baumgartner RN, Koehler KM, Gallagher D, Romero L, Heymsfield SB, Ross RR, Garry PJ, Lindeman RD. 1998. Epidemiology of sarcopenia among the elderly in New Mexico. *Am J Epidemiol* 147(8):755–763.

Campbell AJ, Robertson MC, Gardner MM, Norton RN, Tilyard MW, Buchner DM. 1997. Randomised controlled trial of a general practice programme of home based exercise to prevent falls in elderly women. *BMJ* 315(7115):1065–1069.

CDC (Centers for Disease Control and Prevention). 2005. Trends in leisure-time physical inactivity by age, sex, and race/ethnicity—United States, 1994–2004. *MMWR* 54(39):991–994.

Colcombe S, Kramer AF. 2003. Fitness effects on the cognitive function of older adults: A meta-analytic study. *Psychol Sci* 14(2):125–130.

Cummings SR, Nevitt MC, Browner WS, Stone K, Fox KM, Ensrud KE, Cauley J, Black D, Vogt TM. 1995. Risk factors for hip fracture in white women. Study of Osteoporotic Fractures Research Group. *N Engl J Med* 332(12): 767–773.

Fiatarone MA, O'Neill EF, Ryan ND, Clements KM, Solares GR, Nelson ME, Roberts SB, Kehayias JJ, Lipsitz LA, Evans WJ. 1994. Exercise training and nutritional supplementation for physical frailty in very elderly people. *N Engl J Med* 330(25):1769–1775.

Fleg JL, Morrell CH, Bos AG, Brant LJ, Talbot LA, Wright JG, Lakatta EG. 2005. Accelerated longitudinal decline of aerobic capacity in healthy older adults. *Circulation* 112(5):674–682.

Frontera WR, Suh D, Krivickas LS, Hughes VA, Goldstein R, Roubenoff R. 2000. Skeletal muscle fiber quality in older men and women. *Am J Physiol Cell Physiol* 279(3):C611–C618.

Goodpaster BH, Park SW, Harris TB, Kritchevsky B, Nevitt M, Schwartz AV, Simonsick EM, Tylavsky FA, Visser M, Newman AB, Health ABC Study. 2006. The loss of skeletal muscle strength, mass, and quality in older adults: The Health, Aging and Body Composition Study. *J Gerontol A Biol Sci Med Sci* 61(10):1059–1064.

Heyn P, Abreu BC, Ottenbacher KJ. 2004. The effects of exercise training on elderly persons with cognitive impairment and dementia: A meta-analysis. *Arch Phys Med Rehabil* 85(10):1694–1704.

Jette, AM, Branch LG. 1981. The Framingham Disability Study: II. Physical disability among the aging. *Am J Public Health* 71(11):1211–1216.

Jette AM, Haley SM, Coster WJ, Kooyoomjian JT, Levenson S, Heeren T, Ashba J. 2002. Late life function and disability instrument: I. Development and evaluation of the disability component. *J Gerontol A Biol Sci Med Sci* 57(4):M209–M216.

Keysor JJ, Jette AM. 2001. Have we oversold the benefit of late-life exercise? *J Gerontol A Biol Sci Med Sci* 56(7):M412–M423.

Kramer AF, Erickson KI, Colcombe SJ. 2006. Exercise, cognition, and the aging brain. *J Appl Physiol* 101(4):1237–1242.

Latham NK, Bennett DA, Stretton CM, Anderson CS. 2004. Systematic review of progressive resistance strength training in older adults. *J Gerontol A Biol Sci Med Sci* 59(1):48–61.

The LIFE Investigators. 2006. Effects of a physical activity intervention on measures of physical performance: Results of the Lifestyles Interventions and Independence for Elders Pilot (LIFE-P) study. *J Gerontol* 61A(11).

Manson JE, Skerrett PJ, Greenland P, VanItallie TB. 2004. The escalating pandemics of obesity and sedentary lifestyle. A call to action for clinicians. *Arch Intern Med* 164(3):249–258.

Metter, EJ, Conwit R, Tobin J, Fozard JL. 1997. Age-associated loss of power and strength in the upper extremities in women and men. *J Gerontol A Biol Sci Med Sci* 52(5):B267–B276.

Metter EJ, Lynch N, Conwit R, Lindle R, Tobin J, Hurley B. 1999. Muscle quality and age: Cross-sectional and longitudinal comparisons. *J Gerontol A Biol Sci Med Sci* 54(5):B207–B218.

Morganti CM, Nelson ME, Fiatarone MA, Dallal GE, Economos CD, Crawford BM, Evans WJ. 1995. Strength improvements with 1 yr of progressive resistance training in older women. *Med Sci Sports Exerc* 27(6):906–912.

Nagi SZ. 1965. Some conceptual issues in disability and rehabilitation. In: Sussman MB. *Sociology and Rehabilitation.* Washington, DC: American Sociological Society.

Nelson ME, Fiatarone MA, Morganti CM, Trice I, Greenberg RA, Evans WJ. 1994. Effects of high intensity strength training on multiple risk factors for osteoporotic fractures. *J Am Med Assoc* 272(24):1909–1914.

Newman AB, Lee JS, Visser M, Goodpaster BH, Kritchevsky SB, Tylavsky FA, Nevitt M, Harris TB. 2005. Weight change and the conservation of lean mass in old age: The Health, Aging and Body Composition Study. *Am J Clin Nutr* 82(4):872–878.

Newman AB, Simonsick EM, Naydeck BL, Boudreau RM, Kritchevsky SB, Nevitt MC, Pahor M, Satterfield S, Brach JS, Studenski SA, Harris TB. 2006. Association of long-distance corridor walk performance with mortality, cardiovascular disease, mobility limitation, and disability. *J Am Med Assoc* 295(17):2018–2026.

Ouellette MM, LeBrasseur NK, Bean JF, Phillips E, Stein J, Frontera WR, Fielding RA. 2004. High-intensity resistance training improves muscle strength, self-reported function, and disability in long-term stroke survivors. *Stroke* 35(6):1404–1409.

Penninx BWJH, Kritchevsky SB, Newman AB, Nicklas BJ, Simonsick EM, Rubin S, Nevitt M, Visser M, Harris T, Pahor M. 2004. Inflammatory markers and incident mobility limitation in the elderly. *J Am Geriatr Soc* 52(7):1105–1113.

Roberts SB, Williamson DF. 2002. Causes of adult weight gain. *J Nutr* 132(12):3824S–3825S.

Sayers SP, Brach JS, Newman AB, Heeren TC, Guralnik JM, Fielding RA. 2004. Use of self-report to predict ability to walk 400 meters in mobility-limited older adults. *J Amer Geriatr Soc* 52(12):2099–2103.

Verbrugge LM, Jette AM. 1994. The disablement process. *Soc Sci Med* 38(1):1–14.

Verghese J. 2006. Cognitive and mobility profile of older social dancers. *J Am Geriatr Soc* 54(8):1241–1244.

Weuve J, Kang JH, Manson JE, Breteler MM, Ware JH, Grodstein F. 2004. Physical activity, including walking, and cognitive function in older women. *J Am Med Assoc* 292(12):1454–1461.

Wolf SL, Barnhart HX, Kutner NG, McNeely E, Coogler C, Xu T. 1996. Reducing frailty and falls in older persons: An investigation of tai chi and computerized balance training. Atlants FICSIT Group. Frailty and injuries: Cooperative studies of intervention techniques. *J Am Geriatr Soc* 44(5):489–497.

7

Physical Activity and Considerations for Persons with Disabilities

This chapter focuses on the evidence of the benefits of physical activity for people with a broad range of disabilities. Introductory information is followed by coverage of physical activity related to seven conditions: spinal cord injury, cerebral palsy, multiple sclerosis, intellectual disabilities, stroke, heart disease, and cancer. The chapter ends with highlights from the group discussion.

CONSIDERATIONS FOR PERSONS WITH DISABILITIES

Presenter: James H. Rimmer

The term *disability* has been defined in many ways. For this meeting, Dr. Rimmer proposed that the term be used to describe people who are generally excluded from studies of physical activity, such as persons with severe back pain, persons using assistive devices, persons with cognitive or sensory deficits, and persons having various comorbidities. This presentation included background information on disabilities in the United States, evidence of associations between physical activity and health outcomes for selected types of disability, and the proposed nature of physical activity guidelines for people with disabilities. Dr. Rimmer took the position that this population group merits special attention because people with disabilities were not addressed in *Physical Activity and Health: A Report of the Surgeon General* (DHHS, 1996).

Background

In the United States, approximately 54 million people report some type of disability. Compared with people without disabilities, more people with disabilities report poor health conditions, and they report more conditions that are chronic as well (as tracked through the 2001–2003 Behavioral Risk Factor Surveillance System [BRFSS]). Persons with disabilities also may experience secondary conditions that may be a direct or indirect consequence of having the disability. Examples of such secondary conditions are pain, fatigue, cardiovascular deconditioning, depression, social isolation, and obesity. The direct medical costs for disability are estimated to be $300 billion per year (IOM, 1997).

It is inappropriate to equate disability with poor health: disability and disease are different concepts. Because data seldom are tracked over time, it is not known to what extent certain disabilities increase the risk of a chronic health condition such as obesity. The prevalence rates of overweight, obesity, and extreme obesity were evaluated among 306 adults (108 men, 198 women) with physical and cognitive disabilities. These rates were compared to the respective prevalence rates among adults in the 1999–2000 National Health and Nutrition Examination Survey (Rimmer and Wang, 2005). Results indicated that the rates of overweight, obesity, and extreme obesity were much higher for persons with disabilities than for the general population. Extreme obesity (BMI > 40 kg/m^2) was nearly four times higher among people with disabilities than in the general population.

Persons with a disability tend to be less fit than the general population. For example, in nine recent studies that measured VO_2 peak in subjects with stroke, reported values were significantly lower than typical values for a population of non-disabled adults of similar age and sex (Chu et al., 2004; Duncan et al., 2003; Fujitani et al., 1999; Kelly et al., 2003; MacKay-Lyons and Makrides, 2002; Macko et al., 2001; Potempa et al., 1995; Rimmer et al., 2000; Rimmer et al., submitted).

Compared with healthy individuals, more persons with disabilities report that they are physically inactive, as tracked through BRFSS. The proportion of smokers is higher among those with disabilities as well.

Emerging Evidence on Physical Activity and Disability

When reviewing evidence concerning effects of physical activity among disabled persons, Dr. Rimmer focused on five different disabilities: spinal cord injuries, cerebral palsy, multiple sclerosis, intellectual disabilities, and stroke.

Effects of Exercise on Persons with Spinal Cord Injury

Muscle strength If there is not complete paralysis (for example, with incomplete spinal cord injury), exercise training generally can produce significant gains in strength in paretic muscles through increased motor unit recruitment (Hicks et al., 2003). In people with complete spinal cord injury, intact muscle groups can be strengthened to be similar to the respective muscles in the general population.

Psychosocial Randomized controlled trials on the psychosocial effects of exercise in spinal cord injury show improvements in depression and lower levels of stress (Ginis et al., 2003; Hicks et al., 2003; Latimer et al., 2004), and they show lower levels of pain (Curtis et al., 1999; Hicks et al., 2003; Latimer et al., 2004; Martin Ginis et al., 2003). Ditor and colleagues (2003) found a strong positive effect of exercise on perceived quality of life, but it declined precipitously upon removal of the treatment, and the pain and stress scores rose substantially.

Effects of Exercise in Persons with Cerebral Palsy

Three relatively recent studies show that resistance training 2 to 3 days per week for 6 to 10 weeks leads to significant improvement in the strength of persons with cerebral palsy (Andersson et al., 2003; Dodd et al., 2002; Taylor et al., 2004). In a systematic review of the effectiveness of strength training for people with cerebral palsy, Dodd et al. (2002) found only one randomized controlled trial. Eight of the 10 empirical studies reported moderate increases in strength, 2 studies reported improvement in general activity, and 1 study reported improvements in self-perception. Notably, in all the studies, the improvements occurred without an increase in spasticity or adverse events.

Effects of Exercise in Persons with Multiple Sclerosis

Of four randomized controlled trials on the effects of exercise in persons with multiple sclerosis, one (Petajan et al., 1996) found significant increases in cardiovascular endurance, strength, body composition, blood lipids, psychosocial parameters, and fatigue. The other three studies (Mostert and Kesselring, 2002; Oken et al., 2004; Surakka et al., 2004) had less favorable findings. All but Mostert and Kesselring (2002), however, found significant improvements in fatigue with exercise.

Effects of Exercise in Persons with Intellectual Disabilities

General Seven of 64 reviewed studies on exercise in persons with intellectual disabilities involved a randomized controlled trial, and 15 involved a controlled (nonrandomized) trial or a single group pre- and post-test. The remaining studies were descriptive. The randomized controlled trials found significant increases in VO_2 peak and in duration, workload, and/or distance. Little or no improvement in body composition was found. Two of the studies showed significant increases in strength, decreased perceived barriers to participation in exercise, and increased outcome expectations in self-efficacy and life satisfaction. One study showed increased walking speed among older persons with intellectual disability.

Down Syndrome In a systematic review of the outcomes of cardiovascular exercise programs for persons with Down syndrome (Dodd and Shields, 2005), the findings generally favored treatment. In a quasi-experimental exercise training study involving 14 adolescents (10 experimental and 4 controls) with Down syndrome, Millar et al. (1993) found no change in VO_2 peak but did report improvements in endurance and physical work capacity.

Effects of Exercise in Persons with Stroke

Studies of the effects of exercise in persons with stroke consistently have demonstrated improvements in VO_2 peak (Chu et al., 2004; Duncan et al., 2003; Fujitani et al., 1999; Macko et al., 2005; Potempa et al., 1995; Rimmer et al., 2000). As noted later by Dr. Macko, however, the fractional utilization of maximal aerobic capacity (%VO_2max) may be a more important measure, indicating increased economy of movement—a very important outcome for people affected by stroke.

Rimmer's group examined dose–response effects of exercise in stroke participants. They tested different intensity levels and different durations of exercise and compared the findings with those of the usual care group, which had improvement in gait as the focus of care. The results are summarized in Table 7-1. Outcomes differed based on the intensity or duration of the exercise. The reasons for differences in health outcomes are not yet well understood.

TABLE 7-1 Dose–Response Effects of Aerobic Exercise in Stroke

Effect	Intensity	Duration	Usual Care
Body mass index	NE	↓	NE
Peak VO_2[a]	↑	↑↑	NE
Total cholesterol	↓	NE	NE
HDL	NE	NE	NE
LDL	↓↓	NE	NE
Triglycerides	↓↓	↓↓	↓↓
Gait speed (m/s)	↑↑	↑↑	↑↑
Barthel Function Index[b]	NE	NE	NE
Fatigue Severity Scale	↓↓	↓↓	NE

NOTES: NE = < 5 percent change; one arrow (↓) represents a 5–10 percent change in the direction shown by the arrow; two arrows (↓↓) represents greater than a 10 percent change in the direction shown by the arrows; HDL = high density lipoprotein; LDL = low density lipoprotein; m/s = meters per second;
[a]VO_2 is a measure of oxygen consumption.
[b]Barthel Function Index is a general measure of performance in activities of daily living.
SOURCE: Adapted from Rimmer et al. (2007) (unpublished data).

Nature of Physical Activity Recommendations for People with Disabilities

Appropriate Exclusion Criteria

The development of appropriate exclusion criteria is a valuable approach to help ensure that exercise is safe for a person with a disability. Dr. Rimmer's group identified the exclusion criteria used in seven studies of persons with stroke in which no major adverse events were reported and noted that careful monitoring is needed. With younger, less disabled groups, risks associated with exercise appear to be typical of the general population.

Individualized, Function-Based Guidelines

Because of variances in the data for the frequency, intensity, and time of physical activity for people with disabilities, Dr. Rimmer expressed that guidelines should be individualized and based on health and function instead of disability. The International Classification of Functioning Disability and Health (WHO, 2001) provides a useful model for developing individualized exercise protocols. This model considers body functions and structures, activities, and participation in general life activities. It also considers environmental factors such as accessibility and personal factors such as motivational level or depression. The National Center on Physical Activity and Disability (www.ncpad.org) has developed an instrument to assess an exercise facility to determine what changes would meet the needs of people with disabilities.

Concluding Remarks

Dr. Rimmer emphasized that appropriate physical activity is safe, effective, and very important for people with disabilities. Current data show improvements in oxygen capacity (VO_2), muscular strength, pain (including wheelchair user's shoulder pain), stress, quality of life, physical function, body composition, blood lipids, gait speed, and fatigue. For safety and effectiveness, physical activity guidelines need to be individualized and based on health and function. Moreover, efforts are needed to provide more accessible facilities and programs in the community so that people with disabilities can engage in physical activities to the extent recommended.

In addition, Dr. Rimmer called for a more scientific approach to addressing specific secondary conditions—an approach that includes looking at specific doses of exercise related to effects on pain, fatigue, deconditioning, and obesity.

DISCUSSION

Special Considerations for Persons with Heart Disease

Discussant: Peter H. Brubaker

Background

Approximately 60 million Americans have heart disease, which is the number one cause of death of U.S. men and women. More than 1 million Americans have a myocardial infarction each year, and about one-third of these are fatal. In addition, approximately 1 million Americans undergo cardiovascular operations and procedures each year (AHA 2005).

Heart failure, largely a disease of the elderly, is a major and growing public health problem in the United States. Approximately 5 million Americans have this condition, and the disease is very costly to manage.

Exercise and the Secondary Prevention of Heart Disease

The evidence clearly points to exercise as an effective intervention for the secondary prevention of heart disease. Taylor and colleagues (2004), in a review of 48 randomized controlled trials of exercise training and 8,940 patients, reported the following benefits of 30- to 40-minute moderate-intensity endurance exercise performed three to four times per week over about 2.5 years:

- Twenty percent reduction in all-cause mortality and 26 percent reduction in cardiac mortality
- Improvements in physical function, blood lipids, systolic blood pressure, and selected psychosocial variables

- Improvements in fibrinolysis, thrombocyte aggregation, endothelial function, and other mechanisms of benefit

Benefits of Endurance Exercise Training in Systolic Heart Failure

Walking or cycling three to five times per week at 40 to 80 percent of peak VO_2 for 8 to 24 weeks has been shown to decrease some symptoms of heart failure and improve exercise tolerance, ventilation, quality of life, and many other markers of health (Pina et al., 2003). Closely supervised endurance exercise has not been shown to have adverse effects in this population. One small study showed that exercise twice weekly for 14 months reduced hospitalization and death (Bellardinelli et al., 1999). Similarly, the ExTraMATCH meta-analysis of persons with systolic heart failure (Piepoli et al., 2004) found that those who participate in an exercise training intervention had a significantly lower risk of dying after about 2 years.

Concluding Remarks

Data that are more definitive will be forthcoming. The large multicenter Heart Failure Action study (an ongoing study) is expected to include more than 2,000 patients, and it will examine the impact of exercise training on heart failure, morbidity, and mortality. Some results are anticipated by 2008.

Exercise Models in Persons with Disability from Stroke

Discussant: Richard F. Macko[1]

Rationale for Physical Activity

Metabolic The metabolic rationale for exercise in the chronic phases of stroke relates to body composition and tissue-level abnormalities. Every stroke patient has hemiparetic muscle atrophy, and strength is related, in part, to the cross-sectional area of the muscle. The quality of the affected

[1]Dr. Macko expressed appreciation to study participants with chronic stroke from Maryland and Tuscany.

muscle also is abnormal and contributes to insulin resistance (Ivey et al., 2006). Dr. Macko estimated that, because of body composition and tissue abnormalities, 80 percent of persons who have had a stroke are in a pre-diabetic state or have type 2 diabetes. Data from the Dutch Transient Ischemic Attack Trial (Vermeer et al., 2006) indicate that impaired glucose tolerance and type 2 diabetes mellitus predict a two- to three-fold increase in risk for a recurrent stroke.

Motor learning Studies have shown that treadmill training with task repetition and progression can have motor benefits: improved interlimb stance:swing ratio (Harris-Love et al., 2001), improved timing quadriceps activation (Harris-Love et al., 2004) (which means that the muscles are responding), and increased corticospinal signal strength to the paretic leg (Forrester et al., 2006) (which means that there is a short-term motor adaptation).

Evidence of Benefits from Controlled Trials

A randomized controlled trial of 6 months of treadmill training in persons with chronic hemiparetic stroke demonstrated significant improvements in VO_2 peak and walking speed and a decrease in the energy cost of walking (Macko et al., 2005). The combination may improve one's ability to perform activities of daily living. Notably, Luft (2005) has shown regions of increased brain activation associated with 6 months of treadmill training. The trial of treadmill training also was shown to reduce the insulin-glucose response to about the same extent as would be expected in an exercise program for persons not affected by stroke (Macko et al., 2005). The set of beneficial changes occurred even many years after the occurrence of the stroke.

This is a new area of study with only one small randomized clinical trial published. Currently, a pilot study of a community-based adaptive physical activity program for chronic stroke is being conducted in Tuscany. The emphasis of this relatively low-cost program is on motor learning for mobility, aerobic training, and socialization. Initial findings are promising in that the program appears to improve function and quality of life and to reduce disability to a clinically meaningful degree.

Concluding Remarks

Dr. Macko summarized the strength of the evidence concerning structured physical activity for persons with stroke as follows:

- *Strong* evidence of improvement in peak cardiorespiratory and muscular fitness
- *Moderate* evidence of improvements in metabolic health, walking function, and bone density
- *Preliminary* evidence of improvement in balance, activities of daily living, quality of life, and mood

Dose–intensity and mechanistic studies would provide information needed to optimize the treatment. Community studies with longitudinal health outcomes are needed.

Evidence on the Health Outcomes of Physical Activity in Cancer Survivors

Discussant: Kerry S. Courneya

Background

In the United States, approximately 1.4 million persons are diagnosed with cancer each year. Because of improved survival rates, cancer survivors comprise a growing subpopulation. Currently, there are about 10 million cancer survivors living in the United States. Both quality of life and survival are important to this group.

During treatments, physical activity-related health outcomes of interest include physical fitness and body composition, physical functioning (especially considering the high proportion of older persons affected by cancer), and acute symptoms such as fatigue, pain, nausea, constipation, sleep problems, neuropathies, depression, anxiety, and cognition. Also of interest is the extent to which physical activity or physical fitness may affect treatment decisions, the ability to withstand and complete intensive treatments, and treatment efficacy. Post-treatment, physical activity-related health outcomes of interest may include chronic symptoms, late-appearing effects (e.g., loss of bone mass, cardiomyopathies, fat gain), recurrence, and mortality.

Conclusions from Recent Systematic Reviews

Over a 3-year period, seven systematic reviews have been published concerning physical activity and cancer outcomes (Conn et al., 2006; Douglas, 2005; Galvao and Newton, 2005; Knols et al., 2005; McNeely et al., 2006; Schmitz et al., 2005; Stevinson et al., 2004). These reviews cover about 30 controlled trials (not all of which were randomized). Dr. Courneya summarized the findings as follows:

Physical activity and physical functioning/quality of life outcomes Physical activity improves fitness, body composition, physical functioning, fatigue, and self-esteem of persons affected by cancer. It does not appear to improve body weight, mood, and emotional well-being. Findings appear stronger in the post-treatment setting than during the cancer treatment. Findings are strongest for breast cancer survivors, the population in which the bulk of research has been conducted.

Physical activity and clinical cancer outcomes It is unknown if physical activity influences treatment decisions, efficacy, or completion rates for persons with cancer. Physical activity has been shown to improve biomarkers such as immune factors and insulin-like growth factors. Several recent studies, including two on colorectal cancer, indicate that a higher level of physical activity after diagnosis is associated with a lower recurrence rate and lower overall mortality.

Concluding Remarks

The methodological quality of the studies of physical activity in cancer survivors is modest but improving. Many cancer survivor groups remain unstudied, and insufficient data are available on many outcomes. Very few data are available on resistance exercise or the optimal exercise prescription for any outcome. No randomized controlled trials have addressed physical activity and cancer recurrence and/or mortality.

Group Discussion

Moderator: Gregory W. Heath

Among the points raised during the discussion period were the following:

- Data are available on benefits of physical activity related to a number of prevalent chronic conditions that were not covered during the workshop, including peripheral arterial disease, kidney transplantation, and pulmonary disease.
- The approach to a physical activity guidelines process that is intended for people with disabilities, as well as the "general population," will be a challenge; but it is important because people with disabilities are a part of the fabric of the United States. A *guideline* may be viewed as a general recommendation as to what should be done, and a *prescription* as the specifics of how to do it. One might consider the approach used in the Dietary Guidelines for Americans 2005, in which adaptations are provided for specific situations or conditions. Consideration also could be given to Canada's model of separate physical activity guidelines for older adults, especially since the proportion of disability is high among older persons. In developing physical activity guidelines, suitable representation of the disability community would be useful.
- Achieving adherence to physical activity interventions has posed a considerable challenge in the United States. In Italy, a socially reinforced community program for persons affected by stroke has achieved a high degree of participation for the past 2 years. The use of behavioral strategies to reinforce longitudinal behavior is promising.

REFERENCES

AHA (American Heart Association). 2005. *Heart and Stroke Statistics—Update.* [Online]. Available: http://www.americanheart.org/ [accessed December 18, 2006].

Andersson C, Grooten W, Hellsten M, Kaping K, Mattsson E. 2003. Adults with cerebral palsy: Walking ability after progressive strength training. *Dev Med Child Neurol* 45(4):220–228.

Belardinelli R, Georgiou D, Cianci G, Purcaro A. 1999. Randomized, controlled trial of long-term moderate exercise training in chronic heart failure: Effects on functional capacity, quality of life, and clinical outcome. *Circulation* 99(9):1173–1182.

Chu KS, Eng JJ, Dawson AS, Harris JE, Oakaplan A, Gylfadottir S. 2004. Water-based exercise for cardiovascular fitness in people with chronic stroke: A randomized controlled trial. *Arch Phys Med Rehabil* 85(6):870–874.

Conn VS, Hafdahl AR, Porock DC, McDaniel R, Nielsen PJ. 2006. A meta-analysis of exercise interventions among people treated for cancer. *Support Care Cancer* 14(7):699–712.

Curtis KA, Tyner TM, Zachary L, Lentell G, Brink D, Didyk T, Gean K, Hall J, Hooper M, Klos J, Lesina S, Pacillas B. 1999. Effect of a standard exercise protocol on shoulder pain in long-term wheelchair users. *Spinal Cord* 37(6):421–429.

DHHS (U.S. Department of Health and Human Services). 1996. *Physical Activity and Health: A Report of the Surgeon General.* Office of the Surgeon General, Atlanta, GA: Centers for Disease Control and Prevention, National Center for Chronic Disease Prevention and Health Promotion. [Online]. Available: http://www.cdc.gov/nccdphp/sgr/pdf/sgrfull.pdf [accessed November 14, 2006].

Ditor DS, Latimer AE, Ginis KA, Arbour KP, McCartney N, Hicks AL. 2003. Maintenance of exercise participation in individuals with spinal cord injury: Effects on quality of life, stress and pain. *Spinal Cord* 41(8):446–450.

Dodd KJ, Taylor NF, Damiano DL. 2002. A systematic review of the effectiveness of strength-training programs for people with cerebral palsy. *Arch Phys Med Rehabil* 83(8):1157–1164.

Dodd KJ, Shields N. 2005. A systematic review of the outcomes of cardiovascular exercise programs for people with Down syndrome. *Arch Phys Med Rehabil* 86(10):2051–2058.

Douglas E. 2005. Exercise in cancer patients. *Phys Ther Rev* 10:71–88.

Duncan P, Studenski S, Richards L, Gollub S, Lai SM, Reker D, Perera S, Yates J, Koch V, Rigler S, Johnson D. 2003. Randomized clinical trial of therapeutic exercise in subacute stroke. *Stroke* 34(9):2173–2180.

Forrester LW, Hanley DF, Macko RF. 2006. Effects of treadmill exercise on transcranial magnetic stimulation-induced excitability to quadriceps after stroke. *Arch Phys Med Rehabil* 87(2):229–234.

Fujitani J, Ishikawa T, Akai M, Kakurai S. 1999. Influence of daily activity on changes in physical fitness for people with post-stroke hemiplegia. *Am J Phys Med Rehabil* 78(6):540–544.

Galvao DA, Newton RU. 2005. Review of exercise intervention studies in cancer patients. *J Clin Oncol* 23(4):899–909.

Ginis KA, Latimer AE, McKechnie K, Ditor DS, McCartney N; Hicks L. 2003. Using exercise to enhance subjective well-being among people with spinal cord injury: The mediating influences of stress and pain. *Rehab Psych* 48(3):157–164.

Harris-Love ML, Forrester LW, Macko RF, Silver KH, Smith GV. 2001. Hemiparetic gait parameters in overground versus treadmill walking. *Neurorehabil Neural Repair* 15(2):105–112.

Harris-Love ML, Macko RF, Whitall J, Forrester LW. 2004. Improved hemiparetic muscle activation in treadmill versus overground walking. *Neurorehabil Neural Repair* 18(3):154–160.

Hicks AL, Martin KA, Ditor DS, Latimer AE, Craven C, Bugaresti J, McCartney N. 2003. Long-term exercise training in persons with spinal cord injury: Effects on strength, arm ergometry performance and psychological well-being. *Spinal Cord* 41(1):34–43.

IOM (Institute of Medicine). 1997. *Enabling America: Assessing the Role of Rehabilitation Science and Engineering.* Washington, DC: National Academy Press.

Ivey FM, Ryan AS, Hafer-Macko CE, Garrity BM, Sorkin JD, Goldberg AP, Macko RF. 2006. High prevalence of abnormal glucose metabolism and poor sensitivity of fasting plasma glucose in the chronic phase of stroke. *Cerebrovasc Dis* 22(5-6):368–371.

Kelly PJ, Furie KL, Shafqat S, Rallis N, Chang Y, Stein J. 2003. Functional recovery following rehabilitation after hemorrhagic and ischemic stroke. *Arch Phys Med Rehabil* 84(7):968–972.

Knols R, Aaronson NK, Uebelhart D, Fransen J, Aufdemkampe G. 2005. Physical exercise in cancer patients during and after medical treatment: A systematic review of randomized and controlled clinical trials. *J Clin Oncol* 23(16):3830–3842.

Latimer AE, Ginis KA, Hicks AL, McCartney N. 2004. An examination of the mechanisms of exercise-induced change in psychological well-being among people with spinal cord injury. *J Rehabil Res Dev* 41(5):643–652.

Luft AR, Forrester L, Macko RF, McCombe-Waller S, Whitall J, Villagra F, Hanley DF. 2005. Brain activation of lower extremity movement in chronically impaired stroke survivors. *NeuroImage* 26(1):184–194.

MacKay-Lyons MJ, Makrides L. 2002. Exercise capacity early after stroke. *Arch Phys Med Rehabil* 83(12):1697–1702.

Macko RF, Smith GV, Dobrovolny CL, Sorkin JD, Goldberg AP, Silver KH. 2001. Treadmill training improves fitness reserve in chronic stroke patients. *Arch Phys Med Rehabil* 82(7):879–884.

Macko RF, Ivey FM, Forrester LW, Hanley D, Sorkin JD, Katzel LI, Silver KH, Goldberg AP. 2005. Treadmill exercise rehabilitation improves ambulatory function and cardiovascular fitness in patients with chronic stroke: A randomized, controlled trial. *Stroke* 36(10):2206–2211.

Martin Ginis, KA, Latimer AE, McKechnie K, Ditor DS, McCartney N, Hicks AL, Bugaresti J, Craven C. 2003. Using physical activity to enhance subjective well-being among people with spinal cord injury: The medicating influence of stress and pain. *Rehabilitation Psychology* 48:157-164.

McNeely ML, Campbell KL, Rowe BH, Klassen TP, Mackey JR, Courneya KS. 2006. Effects of exercise on breast cancer patients and survivors: A systematic review and meta-analysis. *Can Med Assoc J* 175(1):34–41.

Millar AL, Fernhall B, Burkett LN. 1993. Effects of aerobic training in adolescents with Down syndrome. *Med Sci Sports Exerc* 25(2):270–274.

Mostert S, Kesselring J. 2002. Effects of a short-term exercise training program on aerobic fitness, fatigue, health perception and activity level of subjects with multiple sclerosis. *Mult Scler* 8(2):161–168.

Oken BS, Kishiyama S, Zajdel D, Bourdette D, Carlsen J, Haas M, Hugos C, Kraemer DF, Lawrence J, Mass M. 2004. Randomized controlled trial of yoga and exercise in multiple sclerosis. *Neurology* 62(11):2058–2064.

Petajan JH, Gappmaier E, White AT, Spencer MK, Mino L, Hicks RW. 1996. Impact of aerobic training on fitness and quality of life in multiple sclerosis. *Ann Neurol* 39(4):432–441.

Piepoli MF, Davos C, Francis DP, Coats AJ, ExTraMATCH Collaborative. 2004. Exercise training meta-analysis of trials in patients with chronic heart failure (ExTraMATCH). *BMJ* 328(7433):189.

Pina IL, Apstein CS, Balady GJ, Belardinelli R, Chaitman BR, Duscha BD, Fletcher BJ, Fleg JL, Myers JN, Sullivan MJ, American Heart Association Committee on exercise, rehabilitation, and prevention. 2003. Exercise and heart failure: A statement from the American Heart Association Committee on exercise, rehabilitation, and prevention. *Circulation* 107(8):1210–1225.

Potempa K, Lopez M, Braun LT, Szidon JP, Fogg L, Tincknell T. 1995. Physiological outcomes of aerobic exercise training in hemiparetic stroke patients. *Stroke* 26(1):101–105.

Rimmer JH, Wang E. 2005. Obesity prevalence among a group of Chicago residents with disabilities. *Arch Phys Med Rehabil* 86(7):1461–1464.

Rimmer JH, Riley B, Creviston T, Nicola T. 2000. Exercise training in a predominantly African-American group of stroke survivors. *Med Sci Sports Exerc* 32(12):1990–1996.

Rimmer JH, Wang E, Nicola T, Rauworth A. 2007. Dose-response effects of aerobic exercise in reducing cardiovascular risk factors and improving health and function in stroke survivors. Unpublished data.

Schmitz KH, Holtzman J, Courneya KS, Masse LC, Duval S, Kane R. 2005. Controlled physical activity trials in cancer survivors: A systematic review and meta-analysis. *Cancer Epidemiol Biomarkers Prev* 14(7):1588–1595.

Stevinson C, Lawlor DA, Fox KR. 2004. Exercise interventions for cancer patients: Systematic review of controlled trials. *Cancer Causes Control* 15(10):1035–1056.

Surakka J, Romberg A, Ruutiainen J, Aunola S, Virtanen A, Karppi SL, Maentaka K. 2004. Effects of aerobic and strength exercise on motor fatigue in men and women with multiple sclerosis: A randomized controlled trial. *Clin Rehabil* 18(7):737–746.

Taylor NF, Dodd KJ, Larkin H. 2004. Adults with cerebral palsy benefit from participating in a strength training programme at a community gymnasium. *Disabil Rehabil* 26(19):1128–1134.

Taylor RS, Brown A, Ebrahim S, Jolliffe J, Noorani H, Rees K, Skidmore B, Stone JA, Thompson DR, Oldridge N. 2004. Exercise-based rehabilitation for patients with coronary heart disease: Systematic review and meta-analysis of randomized controlled trials. *Am J Med* 116(10):682–692.

Vermeer SE, Sandee W, Algra A, Koudstaal PJ, Kappelle LJ, Dippel DW; Dutch TIA Trial Study Group. 2006. Impaired glucose tolerance increases stroke risk in nondiabetic patients with transient ischemic attack or minor ischemic stroke. *Stroke* 37(6):1413–1417.

WHO (World Health Organization). 2001. *International Classification of Functional Disability and Health*. Geneva, Switzerland: WHO.

8

Closing Session

Dr. Haskell moderated the closing session of the workshop. Moderators of the earlier sessions (Drs. Morrow, Dishman, Brubaker, Macera, Freedson, Nelson, and Heath) provided summaries of the information presented, focusing on the nature, level, and strength of the evidence. A group discussion followed, and then Dr. Haskell provided an overall summary. This chapter integrates presentations made during the closing session. It covers risk reduction for a broad range of health conditions and selected populations, risk–benefit considerations of physical activity, and issues raised during the meeting. It also provides a summary of the final group discussion. The chapter concludes with closing remarks made by Dr. Haskell and RADM Penelope Slade Royall.

SUMMARY OF PLENARY SESSIONS

Physical Activity and Risk Reduction

Adults

Much evidence was presented that physical activity reduces the risk of developing many health conditions. Dr. Morrow illustrated this point with a graph such as that shown in Figure 8-1—a graph in which the specific risk could be any one of many adverse health conditions, including cardiovascular disease, type 2 diabetes, osteoporosis, and many other conditions. This prototype graph is characterized by a large decrease in risk when the physical activity level increases from sedentary to moderate, and a further but smaller decrease in risk when the physical activity

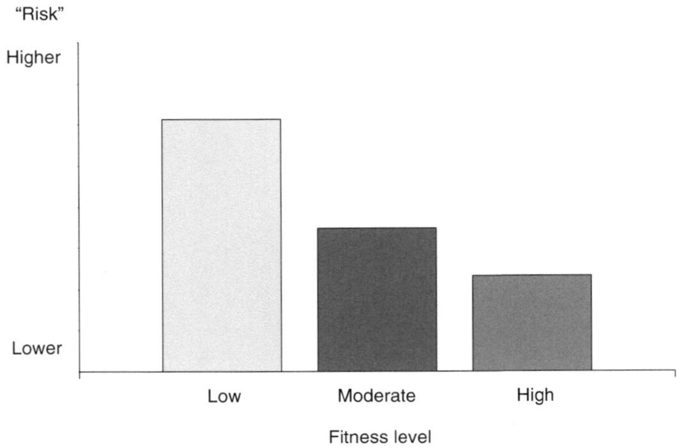

FIGURE 8-1 A representation of the typical relationship between physical activity or fitness level and risk.
NOTE: This general relationship appears to be applicable to the risk of mortality, cardiovascular disease, hypertension, stroke, metabolic disorders, type 2 diabetes mellitus, impaired bone health, impaired mental health status, impaired cognitive ability, some types of cancer, and impaired joint health. The general relationship appears to hold for males, females, persons in different age groups, persons with disabilities, and persons of different racial/ethnic groups.
SOURCE: Morrow (2006).

level increases from moderate to active. Regardless of the morbidity, mortality, or population group (with few exceptions), the evidence shows that those who are more physically active, get more exercise, or are more fit have lower risk. All types of physical activity seem to reduce health risks, and the greater the amount of physical activity—the more fit a person is—the lower the health risks, and one's quality of life is better.

Dr. Haskell summarized the amount and strength of the evidence relating physical activity to selected outcomes for unspecified demographic groups as shown in Table 8-1. *Strength* refers to both quality of data and the magnitude of the association observed. For example, a large effect adds to the strength of the data from an observational study, which ordinarily is viewed as of lower quality than a randomized controlled trial.

TABLE 8-1 Summary of the Amount and Strength of Available Data Relating Physical Activity to Selected Outcomes, Unspecified Demographic Groups

Outcome	Amount[a]	Strength[b]
All-cause mortality	1	1
Major Diseases		
Coronary heart disease	1	1
Cardiovascular disease	1	1
Type 2 diabetes mellitus	1	1
Cancer: colon and breast	1	2
Other cancer sites	2	3
Musculoskeletal		
Muscle quality[c]	1	1
Muscle mass/sarcopenia[d]	1	1
Bone health (osteoporosis)	2	1
Osteoarthritis of knee and hip	2	3
Mental and Neurological Conditions		
Depression	1	1
Anxiety	1	2
Sleep quality	2	1
Alzheimer's disease	2	2
Chronic fatigue syndrome	2	2
Parkinson's disease	3	3
Weight-Related Conditions		
Prevention of weight regain	2	1
Contribution to long-term weight loss	1	2
Metabolic syndrome	2	1
Prevention of unhealthy weight gain	2	2

NOTE: Ratings are approximate; they are not based on a systematic review of the evidence and do not represent a conclusion or consensus reached at this Institute of Medicine workshop.
[a]1 = considerable data; 2 = some data; 3 = limited data.
[b]1 = high; 2 = moderate; 3 = low.
[c]Applies to aerobic and resistance activity.
[d]Applies to resistance activity.

Dr. Haskell commented that, simply in terms of cardiovascular disease and type 2 diabetes, the evidence on benefit from physical activity could be considered sufficient to justify new guidelines and that the evidence of benefit for a number of other conditions also is strong. Comments from other moderators highlighted type 2 diabetes, selected mental and neurological diseases, and weight-related conditions as conditions for which there is sufficient evidence of benefit.

Type 2 diabetes Dr. Dishman noted that strong evidence from observational studies and randomized controlled trials indicates that moderate to vigorous physical activity is associated with a reduced risk of developing type 2 diabetes, even among persons with impaired glucose tolerance, and that the effects usually are independent of weight loss. Moreover, some evidence indicates that physical activity and/or cardiorespiratory fitness favorably modifies cardiovascular events and mortality among persons with type 2 diabetes. Regular physical activity also favorably affects key features of the metabolic syndrome. Chronic effects of exercise include increased insulin sensitivity and responsiveness; improvements in other factors related to glucose use and storage, body fat, skeletal muscle, and lipemic control; and the reduction of comorbidities such as hypertension and systemic inflammation.

Mental and neurological diseases Dr. Dishman summarized that there clearly is a sufficient amount and strength of evidence to justify a systematic review of major depression, some anxiety and sleep disorders, self-esteem, selected features of cognitive function, and chronic pain (data not presented earlier due to lack of time). Evidence to judge dose–response is quite limited and mixed and will require systematic review. Dr. Dishman supplemented earlier presentations by pointing out the availability of a large body of evidence on mechanisms for cognitive and emotional responses to physical activity. Examples include the summary on the neurobiology of exercise by Dishman et al. (2006), studies of exercise and neural plasticity (Anderson et al., 1996; Ang et al., 2003; Black et al., 1990; Carro et al., 2001; Cotman and Berchtold, 2002; Stummer et al., 1994; van Praag et al., 1999, 2005), and studies on the brain–behavior effects of physical activity (Chambliss et al., 2004; Dishman, 1997, Dishman et al., 1997; Greenwood et al., 2003; Russo-Neustadt et al., 2001; van Hoomissen et al., 2003; 2004; Yoo et al., 2000). However, the evidence is almost entirely from animal studies. This is a highly promising emerging area of study.

Weight-related conditions Dr. Brubaker noted that the increase in obesity rates has been accompanied by an increase in so-called unsuccessful attempts at weight loss. Nonetheless, evidence appears to be sufficient to support roles of physical activity for weight loss, the maintenance of weight loss, and the prevention of weight gain. Notably, a clinically significant weight loss of approximately 5 percent of body weight generally represents less weight loss than would be calculated based on energy balance models and much less than the client expects. Dr. Brubaker addressed the difference in the amount of extra energy an individual may need to expend for different purposes: 700 to 1,000 kcal per *week* to prevent inappropriate weight gain versus 500 or 700 kcal per *day* (more than 2,000 kcal per week) to achieve weight loss and/or maintenance of weight loss. He pointed out that these estimates of energy expenditure may need careful consideration in the development of realistic guidelines. Men appear to respond to physical activity interventions with more weight loss than do women. The mechanisms underlying this gender difference are unclear and warrant further investigation. Although not all people respond to physical activity with weight loss, physical activity produces a variety of other health benefits (see above) *independent* of weight loss.

Children and Youth

Table 8-2 summarizes the information about evidence relating physical activity to outcomes for youth. Very little evidence is available about dose–response. A summary of comments from Dr. Freesdon follows.

Children and youth are basically healthy. Regular physical activity results in some improvements in the aerobic fitness and strength of healthy children and adolescents, but improvements in blood pressure and metabolic indicators are observed only in children with compromised health. Weight-bearing exercise has beneficial effects on bone, especially in prepubertal children. The need for different types of physical activity varies with age. Physical inactivity and sedentary behaviors are highly prevalent and merit further attention.

TABLE 8-2 Summary of the Amount and Strength of the Available Data Relating Physical Activity to Selected Outcomes for Children and Youth

Outcome	Amount[a]	Strength[b]
Fitness: strength and endurance	1	1
Skeletal health	2	2
Blood pressure in hypertensive youth	2	2
Weight loss in overweight/obesity	2	2
Metabolic syndrome factors	3	2
High-density lipoprotein cholesterol	2	3
Behavioral outcomes	2	3
Academic performance	2	3
Type 2 diabetes	4	NA

NOTE: Ratings are approximate. They are not based on a comprehensive review of the evidence and do not represent a conclusion or consensus reached at this Institute of Medicine workshop.
[a]1 = considerable data; 2 = some data; 3 = limited data; 4 = very limited data.
[b]1 = high; 2 = moderate; 3 = low.
NA = not applicable.

Pregnant Women

Physical activity appears to benefit women both during pregnancy and the postpartum period. Regular physical activity may lower one's risk for gestational diabetes.

Older Persons

Considerable evidence points to the benefits of physical activity among persons ages 65 years and older, as shown in Table 8-3. Highlights of the comments made by Dr. Nelson appear below.

Chronic illness Most chronic illnesses and other conditions place the greatest burden on older adults. The most notable of these are heart disease, type 2 diabetes, osteoporosis, specific cancers, cognitive impairment, depression, and sleep problems. Evidence indicates that physical activity reduces the risk of developing many of these conditions and helps control signs and symptoms once a condition is established.

TABLE 8-3 Summary of the Amount and Strength of the Available Data Relating Physical Activity to Selected Outcomes, Persons Age 65 Years and Older

Outcome	Amount[a]	Strength[b]
Coronary heart disease and cardiovascular disease	1	1
Diabetes mellitus	1	1
Osteoporosis	1	1
Sarcopenia (muscle wasting)	1	1
Fitness: endurance, strength, balance	1	1
Activities of daily living	1	1
Sleep quality	2	1
Cognitive function	1	2
Fall prevention	2	2
Disability	2	3

NOTE: Ratings are approximate. They are not based on a comprehensive review of the evidence and do not represent a conclusion or consensus reached at this Institute of Medicine workshop. Wide variations in older persons' ability to perform and in their response to activity call for caution in developing physical activity recommendations.
[a]1 = considerable data; 2 = some data; 3 = limited data; 4 = very limited data.
[b]1 = high; 2 = moderate; 3 = low.

Physiological markers A large body of literature addresses physiological markers. It includes strong evidence both from observational and intervention studies that physical activity improves muscle mass and strength, bone, balance, and functional performance. Aerobic capacity declines in older adults; however, physically active older adults have higher oxygen capacity (VO_2) than sedentary peers and some have higher VO_2 than sedentary younger persons. A wide variety of physical activities improve muscle mass and strength, bone, balance, and functional performance.

Falls prevention A moderate amount of moderate to strong evidence addresses physical activity and the prevention of falls. Targeted physical activity interventions—especially those with a balance component—reduce falls in community-dwelling frail elders.

Disability Physical activity influences all segments of the path to disability among older persons. High body fat content and poor quality of muscle increase the risk of disability. Well-designed randomized controlled trials are needed to better establish how various exercise regimens affect the incidence of disability and hospitalization in older persons at high risk of becoming frail.

Special considerations Consideration of the evidence relating to physical activity in older adults merits attention to their great heterogeneity (many are in good health), body weight that is in flux, effects of intercurrent illness, and specific medical conditions.

Persons with Disabilities or Selected Chronic Conditions

According to Dr. Heath, strong evidence documents that individuals with disabilities have the capacity to adapt to increased levels of physical activity and that increased levels of physical activity can produce the following effects:

- Improved cardiorespiratory fitness
- Increases in muscular strength and endurance
- Improved metabolic health (particularly carbohydrate and lipid metabolism)
- Improved psychosocial status
- Improved health-related quality of life

Among persons with coronary heart disease, physical activity-based cardiac rehabilitation reduces all-cause mortality and cardiac mortality. A moderate amount of evidence documents that increases in physical activity lead to beneficial changes in body composition, improved physical functioning, decreased fatigue, improved cardiovascular disease risk profile, and improved ventilation and decreased dyspnea (shortness of breath) among persons with heart failure and chronic obstructive pulmonary disease.

Insufficient evidence is available to determine whether or not increases in physical activity influence treatment decisions, improve selected biomarkers, lead to lower recurrence rates and longer survival among cancer survivors, prevent and/or reduce the occurrence of secondary conditions, alter underlying disease processes, decrease disability, or improve function.

Physical Activity and Risk—Maximizing Benefits

According to Dr. Macera, a large body of literature documents the risk of physical activity-related injuries. Strong evidence indicates that it is possible to reduce injury risks that otherwise may deter individuals from being active. A suggested approach in developing guidelines is to consider evidence of how to maximize the benefits of physical activity while minimizing the risks.

Strong evidence is available to support the following points regarding physical activity and risk:

Injury Risk

- Any movement increases the risk for injury.
- Activities such as running or vigorous sports are associated with more injuries than are such activities as walking.
- Recreational and competitive runners have a high prevalence of injury (average about 45 percent per year).
- Higher amounts of past physical activity protect against current injury.
- Higher levels of physical fitness protect against injury.
- Active individuals may have lower occurrence of overall injury.
- A sedentary lifestyle is associated with an elevated risk of injury when actually engaging in physical activity.
- In military settings with a standard exercise training protocol, women have higher injury rates than men; this effect diminishes when adjusted for fitness.
- Extremes of flexibility (too loose or too tight) are associated with injury risk among military subjects.

Cardiovascular Risk

- Sudden cardiac arrest is more common during exercise than during sedentary activities.
- The risk of cardiovascular adverse effects goes down with habitual activity.

- The relative risk of sudden death during vigorous exercise is lowest among people who exercise regularly (e.g., $\geq$ 5 times per week).

Weaker evidence suggests that smoking may be associated with an elevated risk of injury and that very high or low body mass index (BMI) may be associated with increased risk.

In general, the database of studies of physical activity and risk is rich, including many diverse settings and populations. Much of the evidence comes from military studies with prescribed training schedules and standard injury assessment procedures. Among the weaknesses of the evidence are a lack of a common injury definition, small sample sizes, and a limited range of ages of subjects. More information is needed on specific injury risks associated with special populations, long-term effects of acute as well as overuse injuries, and effects of excessive physical activity on eating disorders and joint problems

In summary, a strong body of evidence about physical activity-related injuries and sudden cardiac events can be evaluated as a component of a process to develop physical activity guidelines. Most modifiable risk factors for injury are related to frequency, intensity, duration, and type of activity. The injury experience of youth, older adults, and those with disabilities merits special attention.

Issues Raised During the Workshop

Over the course of the workshop, several issues were raised that warrant further attention. Among these issues were those relating to improving measurement (including the use of more objective measures of physical activity), consideration of both acute and chronic effects of physical activity, the scope and role of biomarkers in assessing benefit, exercise as medicine, message confusion, validity, and dose–response.

According to Dr. Morrow, it can be useful to view physical activity as a medicine—one that has preventive, therapeutic, and treatment characteristics. Physical activity can help people stay healthy, and it can help people with many types of health problems become healthier.

With regard to message confusion, the following words may have different meanings to different people: *light*, *moderate*, *brisk*, *heavy*, *vigorous*, *exercise*, *physical activity*, *typical*, *most*, and *average*.

Dr. Morrow pointed out that the evidence on benefits of physical activity appears to have external validity because it generalizes to mortality and to a wide variety of morbidities, different populations, and activity styles. Internal validity is strongly suggested by the convergence of findings from different types of studies.

When examining dose–response data, consideration may be given to the duration of the physical activity bout, the intensity and frequency of the bouts, the number of kilocalories used, and/or the total volume of exercise. Several participants suggested giving consideration to the least amount of physical activity that will produce benefit.

DISCUSSION

Before closing the session, moderator William Haskell invited attendees to share new information about outcomes already discussed as well as new outcomes that they wanted to place on the record. The statements made should not be interpreted as representing recommendations or the consensus of the workshop.

Physical Activity in Diverse Racial and Ethnic Groups

Several examples were given of comparable results in studies that involved two or more racial/ethnic groups. Such studies include the Diabetes Prevention Program (DPP Research Group, 2002), and the response of bone to an exercise intervention (MacKelvie et al., 2002).

Health Benefits of Physical Activity for Children and Adolescents

Preschool children, in particular, are an understudied group. The terms *physical activity* and *fitness* are not interchangeable in children and youth in the way they may be used for adults. Work by Dr. Catrine Tudor-Locke et al. (2006) and colleagues (Flohr et al., 2006) address the correspondence of a recommended number of steps per day for children and adolescents with the guideline to obtain 60 minutes of physical activity daily.

Evidence Related to Additional Health Conditions

A large bibliography that includes references on physical activity and pain soon will be available through the American Pain Society. The occurrence of fibromyalgia appears to be increasing and merits attention.

Benefits of Specific Types of Physical Activity

Considerable discussion occurred in response to a question about evidence to support the development of guidelines that address specific *types* of physical activity. For example, what health-related conditions are likely to be most affected by resistance training, and what is the strength of the evidence? Useful sources of information include work by the following:

- Cussler et al. (2003, 2005) and Lohman et al. (1995) regarding strength training and bone
- Sigal (2004) regarding a trial of aerobic and resistance exercise related to diabetes
- FitzGerald (2004) regarding strength training and all-cause mortality
- Meyer (2006) regarding strength training in patients with chronic congestive heart failure
- Singh et al. (2005) regarding strength training and depression in older persons
- Castaneda et al. (2002) regarding strength training in Hispanics with diabetes
- Faigenbaum et al. (2001) and colleagues (Hoffman et al., 2005) regarding children and youth

Balance training and multimodal interventions—not just resistance training—should be considered. However, relatively little evidence appears to be available that compares effects of different types of exercise.

Interrelationships of Physical Activity and Nutrition

Emphasis was placed on considering diet as well as physical activity with regard to weight-related benefits. A meta-analysis conducted by

Miller and colleagues (1997) and the report by Saris et al. (2003) from the International Obesity Taskforce provide pertinent information on the effects of physical activity on weight management. Physical activity and nutrition interact in many other conditions as well. Examples include the acquisition of lean body mass, diabetes mellitus, bone health, and metabolic syndrome.

Strategy for Interpreting the Scientific Evidence

Dr. Pate advised the application of a conservative strategy in interpreting the literature, and the value of this approach was reinforced by Dr. Haskell. There is great variability in the strength of the evidence on physical activity in relation to benefit and risk. The strong evidence that has accumulated since prior efforts at guidelines development for three or four of the major chronic disease conditions in adults can serve as a basis for further development of such evidence-informed guidelines. Several persons pointed out the importance of developing clear evidence-based messages.

CONCLUDING REMARKS

Overall Summary

Presenter: William Haskell

With the substantial decrease in the amount of daily activity required for living among the U.S. population, *physical inactivity* has become a major public health problem. The problem continues to grow. Nonetheless, the United States currently lacks up-to-date, comprehensive physical activity guidelines for promoting health. Lack of such guidelines is a deterrent to the implementation of an effective national physical activity plan. Scientific data collected over the past five or six decades strongly support numerous health benefits of a physically active lifestyle throughout the life span. The nature of the evidence that can be accumulated regarding behaviors—in this case, physical activity behaviors—makes it essential to take into account the strength of a variety of types of evidence (see Figure 1-1 in Chapter 1). The dose–response data that were presented indicate that the development of new or comprehensive guidelines based on such new evidence would be feasible. The evidence presented at the workshop clearly indicates that the large volume of high-quality data—much of it recent—could inform new physical activity guidelines.

Next Steps

Presenter: RADM Penelope Slade-Royall

On behalf of the U.S. Department of Health and Human Services (DHHS), RADM Royall expressed thanks to all who took part in the workshop and provided outstanding information for the department's consideration. She and her colleagues would consider the evidence presented at this workshop and make recommendations to the Secretary of DHHS. Collaborators include Melissa Johnson from the President's Council on Physical Fitness and Sports, CAPT Richard Troiano from the Office of Disease Prevention and Health Promotion of the Office of Public Health and Science, and Harold W. (Bill) Kohl III from the Centers for Disease Control and Prevention. A decision about initiating the process of developing physical activities guidelines is expected to be released soon.

REFERENCES

Anderson BJ, Alcantara AA, Greenough WT. 1996. Motor-skill learning: Changes in synaptic organization of the rat cerebellar cortex. *Neurobiol Learn Mem* 66(2):221–229.

Ang ET, Wong PT, Moochhala S, Ng YK. 2003. Neuroprotection associated with running: Is it a result of increased endogenous neurotrophic factors? *Neuroscience* 118(2):335–345.

Black JE, Isaacs KR, Anderson BJ, Alcantara AA, Greenough WT. 1990. Learning causes synaptogenesis, whereas motor activity causes angiogenesis, in cerebellar cortex of adult rats. *Proc Natl Acad Sci USA* 87(14):5568–5572.

Carro E, Trejo JL, Busiguina S, Torres-Aleman I. 2001. Circulating insulin-like growth factor I mediates the protective effects of physical exercise against brain insults of different etiology and anatomy. *J Neurosci* 21(15):5678–5684.

Castaneda C, Layne J, Munoz-Orians L, Gordon P, Walsmith J, Foldvari M, Roubenoff R, Tucker K, Nelson M. 2002. High-intensity progressive resistance exercise training in Hispanic older adults with type 2 diabetes: A randomized controlled trial. *Diabetes Care* 25(12):2335–2341.

Chambliss HO, Van Hoomissen JD, Holmes PV, Bunnell BN, Dishman RK. 2004. Effects of chronic activity wheel running and imipramine on masculine copulatory behavior after olfactory bulbectomy. *Physiol Behav* 82(4): 593–600.

Cotman CW, Berchtold NC. 2002. Exercise: A behavioral intervention to enhance brain health and plasticity. *Trends Neurosci* 25(6):295–301.

Cussler EC, Lohman TG, Going SB, Houtkooper LB, Metcalfe LL, Flint-Wagner HG, Harris RB, Teixeira PJ. 2003. Weight lifted in strength training predicts bone change in postmenopausal women. *Med Sci Sports Exerc* 35(1):10–17.

Cussler EC, Going SB, Houtkooper LB, Stanford VA, Blew RM, Flint-Wagner HG, Metcalfe LL, Choi JE, Lohman TG. 2005. Exercise frequency and calcium intake predict 4-year bone changes in postmenopausal women. *Osteoporos Int* 16(12):2129–2141

Dishman RK. 1997. Brain monoamines, exercise, and behavioral stress: Animal models. *Med Sci Sports Exerc* 29(1):63–74.

Dishman RK, Renner KJ, Youngstedt SD, Reigle TG, Bunnell BN, Burke KA, Yoo HS, Mougey EH, Meyerhoff JL. 1997. Activity wheel running reduces escape latency and alters brain monoamine levels after footshock. *Brain Res Bull* 42(5):399–406.

Dishman RK, Berthoud HR, Booth FW, Cotman CW, Edgerton VR, Fleshner MR, Gandevia SC, Gomez-Pinilla F, Greenwood BN, Hillman CH, Kramer AF, Levin BE, Moran TH, Russo-Neustadt AA, Salamone JD, Van Hoomissen JD, Wade CE, York DA, Zigmond MJ. 2006. Neurobiology of exercise. *Obesity (Silver Spring)* 14(3):345–356.

DPP (Diabetes Prevention Program) Research Group. 2002. The Diabetes Prevention Program (DPP): Description of lifestyle intervention. *Diabetes Care* 25(12):2165–2171.

Faigenbaum AD, Loud RL, O'Connell J, Glover S, O'Connell J, Westcott WL. 2001. Effects of different resistance training protocols on upper-body strength and endurance development in children. *J Strength Cond Res* 15(4):459–465.

FitzGerald SJ, Barlow CE, Kampert JB, Morrow JR Jr, Jackson AW, Blair SN. 2004. Muscular fitness and all-cause mortality: Prospective observations. *J Phys Activ Health* 1:7–18.

Flohr JA, Todd MK, Tudor-Locke C. 2006. Pedometer-assessed physical activity in young adolescents. *Res Q Exerc Sport* 77(3):309–315.

Greenwood BN, Foley TE, Day HE, Campisi J, Hammack SH, Campeau S, Maier SF, Fleshner M. 2003. Freewheel running prevents learned helplessness/behavioral depression: Role of dorsal raphe serotonergic neurons. *J Neurosci* 23(7):2889–2898.

Hoffman JR, Kang J, Faigenbaum AD, Ratamess NA. 2005. Recreational sports participation is associated with enhanced physical fitness in children. *Res Sports Med* 13(2):149–161.

Lohman T, Going S, Pamenter R, Hall M, Boyden T, Houtkooper L, Ritenbaugh C, Bare L, Hill A, Aickin M. 1995. Effects of resistance training on regional and total bone mineral density in premenopausal women: A randomized prospective study. *J Bone Miner Res* 10(7):1015–1024.

MacKelvie KJ, McKay HA, Petit MA, Moran O, Khan KM. 2002. Bone mineral response to a 7-month randomized controlled, school-based jumping intervention in 121 prepubertal boys: Associations with ethnicity and body mass index. *J Bone Miner Res* 17(5):834–844.

Meyer K. 2006. Resistance exercise in chronic heart failure—Landmark studies and implications for practice. *Clin Invest Med* 29(3):166–169.

Miller WC, Koceja DM, Hamilton EJ. 1997. A meta-analysis of the past 25 years of weight loss research using diet, exercise or diet plus exercise intervention. *Int J Obes Relat Metab Disord* 21(10):941–947.

Morrow J. 2006. *Physical activity, health promotion, and chronic disease prevention.* Presentation at the Institute of Medicine Workshop on the Adequacy of Evidence for Physical Activity Guidelines Development. Washington, DC. October 23.

Russo-Neustadt A, Ha T, Ramirez R, Kesslak JP. 2001. Physical activity-antidepressant treatment combination: Impact on brain-derived neurotrophic factor and behavior in an animal model. *Behav Brain Res* 120(1):87–95.

Saris WH, Blair SN, van Baak MA, Eaton SB, Davies PS, Di Pietro L, Fogelholm M, Rissanen A, Schoeller D, Swinburn B, Tremblay A, Westerterp KR, Wyatt H. 2003. How much physical activity is enough to prevent unhealthy weight gain? Outcome of the IASO 1st Stock Conference and consensus statement. *Obes Res* 4(2):101–114.

Sigal RJ, Kenny GP, Wasserman DH, Castaneda-Sceppa C. 2004. Physical activity/exercise and type 2 diabetes. *Diabetes Care* 27(10):2518–2539.

Singh NA, Stavrinos TM, Scarbek Y, Galambos G, Liber C, Fiatarone-Singh MA. 2005. A randomized controlled trial of high versus low intensity weight training versus general practitioner care for clinical depression in older adults. *J Gerontol A Biol Sci Med Sci* 60(6):768–776.

Stummer W, Weber K, Tranmer B, Baethmann A, Kempski O. 1994. Reduced mortality and brain damage after locomotor activity in gerbil forebrain ischemia. *Stroke* 25(9):1862–1869.

Tudor-Locke C, Lee SM, Morgan CF, Beighle A, Pangrazi RP. 2006. Children's pedometer-determined physical activity during the segmented school day. *Med Sci Sports Exerc* 38(10):1732–1738.

Van Hoomissen JD, Chambliss HO, Holmes PV, Dishman RK. 2003. Effects of chronic exercise and imipramine on mRNA for BDNF after olfactory bulbectomy in rat. *Brain Res* 974(1-2):228–235.

Van Hoomissen JD, Holmes PV, Zellner AS, Poudevigne A, Dishman RK. 2004. Effects of beta-adrenoreceptor blockade during chronic exercise on contextual fear conditioning and mRNA for galanin and brain-derived neurotrophic factor. *Behav Neurosci* 118(6):1378–1390.

van Praag H, Christie BR, Sejnowski TJ, Gage FH. 1999. Running enhances neurogenesis, learning, and long-term potentiation in mice. *Proc Natl Acad Sci USA* 96(23):13427–13431.
van Praag H, Shubert T, Zhao C, Gage FH. 2005. Exercise enhances learning and hippocampal neurogenesis in aged mice. *J Neurosci* 25(38):8680–8685.
Yoo HS, Tackett RL, Bunnell BN, Crabbe JB, Dishman RK. 2000. Antidepressant-like effects of physical activity vs. imipramine: Neonatal clomipramine model. *Psychobiology* 28(4):540–549.

A

Workshop Agenda

Institute of Medicine Workshop on the Adequacy of Evidence for Physical Activity Guidelines Development
October 23–24, 2006
Washington, DC

October 23rd
National Academy of Sciences Building
2100 C Street, N.W.

October 24th
Keck Center of The National Academies
500 Fifth Street, N.W.

October 23, 2006 **National Academy of Sciences Building**

8:30 am–9:30 am
Opening Session

8:30 am–8:40 am
Welcome

Linda Meyers, Food and Nutrition Board, Institute of Medicine

RADM Penelope Slade Royall, Office of Disease Prevention and Health Promotion, U.S. Department of Health and Human Services

8:40 am–9:00 am
Workshop Purpose and Scope
William Haskell, Chair, IOM Planning Committee and Stanford University Prevention Research Center

9:00 am–9:30 am
State of the Nation Relative to Physical Activity Recommendations
Russell Pate, University of South Carolina

9:30 am–10:30 am
Plenary Session 1

Physical Activity, Health Promotion, and Chronic Disease Prevention
Moderator: *James Morrow,* University of North Texas

9:30 am–10:00 am
All-Cause Mortality, Cardiovascular Disease, and Cancer
Steven Blair, University of South Carolina

10:00 am–10:30 am
Bone, Joint, and Muscle Health and Performance
Wendy Kohrt, University of Colorado

10:45 am–12:30 pm
Plenary Session 2

Physical Activity, Health Promotion, and Chronic Disease Prevention *(continued)*
Moderator: *Rodney Dishman,* University of Georgia

10:45 am–11:15 am
Mental and Neurological Health
Patrick O'Connor, University of Georgia

11:15 am–11:45 am
Diabetes and Other Metabolic Disorders
Judith Regensteiner, University of Colorado

11:45 am–12:30 pm

Discussion

Discussants:

Laurie Goodyear, Harvard Medical School
Bradley Hatfield, University of Maryland (slides presented by *Rodney Dishman*)

Other Panelists:

James Morrow, University of North Texas
Rodney Dishman, University of Georgia
Wendy Kohrt, University of Colorado
Patrick O'Connor, University of Georgia
Judith Regensteiner, University of Colorado

1:30 pm–2:30 pm
Plenary Session 3

Physical Activity, Obesity, and Weight Management
Moderator: *Peter Brubaker,* Wake Forest University

1:30 pm–2:00 pm
Effects of Physical Activity on Weight Gain, Weight Loss, and Weight Loss Maintenance

Joseph Donnelly, University of Kansas

2:00 pm–2:30 pm
Discussion

Discussants:

Andrew Goldberg, Baltimore VA Medical Center
Glenn Gaesser, University of Virginia

Other Panelists:

Peter Brubaker, Wake Forest University
Joseph Donnelly, University of Kansas

2:30 pm–3:30 pm
Plenary Session 4

Physical Activity and Risk—Maximizing Benefits
Moderator: *Caroline Macera,* San Diego State University

2:30 pm–2:50 pm
Risks of Musculoskeletal Injury
Bruce Jones, U.S. Army Center for Health Promotion and Preventive Medicine, Aberdeen

2:50 pm–3:10 pm
Cardiovascular Disease and Related Risks
David Siscovick, University of Washington

3:10 pm–3:30 pm
Discussion

Discussants:
Jennifer Hootman, Centers for Disease Control and Prevention
William Garrett Jr., Duke University

Other Panelists:
Caroline Macera, San Diego State University
Bruce Jones, U.S. Army Center for Health Promotion and Preventive Medicine, Aberdeen
David Siscovick, University of Washington

3:45 pm–6:00 pm
Plenary Session 5

Special Considerations for Children and Youth, Pregnant and Postpartum Women, and Older Adults

Special Considerations for Children and Youth, Pregnant and Postpartum Women
Moderator: *Patty Freedson,* University of Massachusetts

3:45 pm–4:15 pm
Physical Activity and Children and Youth
Robert Malina, Tarleton State University

4:15 pm–5:00 pm
Discussion

Discussants:
Russell Pate, University of South Carolina
Heather McKay, University of British Columbia
James Pivarnik, Michigan State University

Other Panelists:

Patty Freedson, University of Massachusetts
Robert Malina, Tarleton State University

Special Considerations for Older Adults
Moderator: *Miriam Nelson,* Tufts University

5:00 pm–5:30 pm
Physical Activity and Older Adults
Roger Fielding, Tufts University

5:30 pm–6:00 pm
Discussion

Discussant:
Anne Newman, University of Pittsburgh

Other Panelists:
Miriam Nelson, Tufts University
Roger Fielding, Tufts University

October 24, 2006
Keck Center of The National Academies

8:30 am–8:45 am
Review of Previous Day's Presentations

8:45 am–10:00 am
Plenary Session 6

Special Considerations *(continued)*
Moderator: *Gregory Heath,* University of Tennessee at Chattanooga

8:45 am–9:15 am
Special Considerations for Persons with Disabilities
James Rimmer, University of Illinois at Chicago

9:15 am–10:00 am
Discussion

Discussants:

Peter Brubaker, Wake Forest University
Kerry Courneya, University of Alberta
Richard Macko, University of Maryland

Other Panelists:

Gregory Heath, University of Tennessee at Chattanooga
James Rimmer, University of Illinois at Chicago

10:30 am–12:45 pm
Overview of Workshop Discussions

10:30 am–11:15 am
Brief Summary of Plenary Sessions by the Moderators

James Morrow, University of North Texas
Rodney Dishman, University of Georgia
Peter Brubaker, Wake Forest University
Caroine Macera, San Diego State University
Patty Freedson, University of Massachusetts
Miriam Nelson, Tufts University
Gregory Heath, University of Tennessee at Chattanooga

11:15 am–12:15 pm
Plenary Discussion Including Comments from Participants
Moderator: *William Haskell,* Chair, IOM Planning Committee and Stanford University Prevention Research Center

12:15 pm–12:45 pm
Summary of Key Elements of Workshop

William Haskell, Chair, IOM Planning Committee and Stanford University Prevention Research Center

12:45 pm–1:00 pm
Concluding Remarks

RADM Penelope Slade Royall, Office of Disease Prevention and Health Promotion, Office of Public Health and Sciences, U.S. Department of Health and Human Services

B

Presenter Biographical Sketches

Steven N. Blair, P.E.D., is a Professor at the Arnold School of Public Health at the University of South Carolina and an Executive Lecturer in the Department of Kinesiology, Health Promotion, and Recreation at the University of North Texas. Dr. Blair also serves an Adjunct Professor at the School of Public Health, University of Texas Health Science Center at Houston, and the College of Education at the University of Houston; and a Benjamin Meaker Fellow at the University of Bristol, England. Dr. Blair's research focuses on the associations between lifestyle and health, with a specific emphasis on exercise, physical fitness, body composition, and chronic disease. Dr. Blair is the recipient of three honorary doctoral degrees—Doctor *Honoris Causa* degree from the Free University in Brussels, Belgium; Doctor of Health Science degree from Lander University; and Doctor of Science *Honoris Causa* from the University of Bristol in the United Kingdom. Dr. Blair is a Fellow of the American College of Epidemiology, Society for Behavioral Medicine, American College of Sports Medicine, American Heart Association, and the American Academy of Kinesiology and Physical Education. He is also a member of the American Epidemiological Society. He was the first president of the National Coalition for Promoting Physical Activity and is a past-president of the American College of Sports Medicine and the American Academy of Kinesiology and Physical Education. Dr. Blair was granted a MERIT Award from the National Institutes of Health (NIH) and is one of the few individuals outside the U.S. Public Health Service to be awarded the Surgeon General's Medallion. He has published widely in the scientific literature and served as the Senior Scientific Editor for the U.S. Surgeon General's Report on Physical Activity and Health.

Peter H. Brubaker, Ph.D., is a Professor in the Department of Health and Exercise Science and Executive Director of the Healthy Exercise and Lifestyle Programs (formerly Cardiac Rehabilitation) at Wake Forest University in Winston-Salem, North Carolina. He is a Fellow of the American College of Sports Medicine and the American Association of Cardiopulmonary Rehabilitation. Dr. Brubaker has published widely in the scientific literature on the topics of exercise physiology and cardiology and he is coauthor of the textbook, *Coronary Artery Disease: Essentials of Prevention and Rehabilitation Programs*. He served as the Clinical Section Editor of the ACSM *Guidelines for Exercise Testing and Prescription* (7th edition). His research and clinical work focus on heart failure exercise physiology and cardiovascular disease prevention and rehabilitation. His current NIH-supported research focuses on the effect of exercise interventions on aging, obesity, and heart failure.

Kerry S. Courneya, Ph.D., is a Professor and Canada Research Chair in Physical Activity and Cancer in the Faculty of Physical Education at the University of Alberta in Edmonton, Canada. He received his B.A. degree and M.A. degree in physical education from the University of Western Ontario in London, Canada, and his Ph.D. in kinesiology from the University of Illinois at Urbana. Dr. Courneya served as an Assistant and Associate Professor at the University of Calgary for five years before moving to the University of Alberta in 1997. Professor Courneya's research program focuses on the role of physical activity in cancer control, including primary prevention, coping with treatments, rehabilitation after treatments, and secondary prevention and survival. His research interests include both the determinants and outcomes of physical activity for cancer control and behavior change interventions. His research has been funded by the National Cancer Institute of Canada, the Canadian Breast Cancer Research Alliance, the NIH, the Lance Armstrong Foundation, the Alberta Heritage Foundation for Medical Research, and the Alberta Cancer Board.

Rodney K. Dishman, Ph.D., is a Professor of Kinesiology and an Adjunct Professor of Psychology at the University of Georgia. In this capacity, he advises graduate students studying exercise neuroscience and interventions to increase physical activity. Dr. Dishman received his Ph.D. at the University of Wisconsin-Madison. His research has focused on the behavioral determinants of physical activity and the neurobiological aspects of mental health outcomes associated with physical activity. His research has been supported by the NIH, the Centers for Disease Control and Prevention (CDC), the American Heart Association (AHA), and the United States Olympic Committee. Dr. Dishman is a Fellow of the American College of Sports Medicine, the American Psychological Association, and the American Academy of Kinesiology and Physical Education. He has served as a consultant on exercise to the NIH, CDC, the Sports Medicine Council for the USOC, and the Olympic Prize subcommittee of the Medical Commission of the International Olympic Committee (IOC). He was one of 22 founding members of the IOC's Olympic Academy of Sport Sciences.

Joseph E. Donnelly, Ed.D., FACSM, is a Professor and Director of the Energy Balance Laboratory and the University of Kansas Center for Physical Activity and Weight Management in Lawrence, Kansas. Dr. Donnelly is the founder and Director of the annual University of Kansas Conference on Prevention and Treatment of Obesity that is attended by 500 health-care providers. His research support derives from NIH, foundation, and industry for a variety of physical activity and nutrition projects that involve both children and adults. He is widely published in the scientific literature and has authored two college textbooks. He was a coauthor for the American College of Sports Medicine (ACSM) Position Paper on Appropriate Strategies for Weight Reduction and Maintenance in Adults. Dr. Donnelly chairs the NIH Psychosocial Risk and Disease Prevention Study Section. He received his Ed.D. from West Virginia University in Morgantown and is a Fellow of ACSM.

Roger A. Fielding, Ph.D., is Director and Scientist I at the Nutrition, Exercise Physiology, and Sarcopenia Laboratory at the Jean Mayer U.S. Department of Agriculture (USDA) Human Nutrition Research Center on Aging and a Professor of Nutrition at the Friedman School of Nutrition Science and Policy at Tufts University in Boston. He also serves as Codirector of the Tufts-New England Medical Center Clinical Research Center. Dr. Fielding's research interests include the examination of the underlying mechanisms that contribute to the age-associated decline in skeletal muscle mass, the resulting impact on function, and the potential role of exercise and other therapeutic interventions on attenuating this process. His research is currently supported by USDA, the National Institute on Aging (NIA), private foundations, and industry. Dr. Fielding served as Chair of the Lifestyle Interventions for Elders (LIFE) Study

Intervention and Operations Committee that oversaw the development of the physical activity interventions for the LIFE Pilot Study. He is Coinvestigator and Chair of the Body Composition Analysis Committee for the NIA-funded "Calerie" (Comprehensive Assessment of Long-term Effects of Reducing Intake of Energy) Trial, and a member of the Physical Dysfunction Committee for the NIA-funded Testosterone Trial Planning Grant. Dr. Fielding is a member of the American College of Sports Medicine, the American Physiological Society, and the National Scientific Advisory Council of the American Federation for Aging Research.

Patty S. Freedson, Ph.D., is a Professor and Chair in the Kinesiology Department at the University of Massachusetts at Amherst. She instructs undergraduate and graduate students in anatomy and physiology, exercise physiology, physiology of training and conditioning, pediatric exercise physiology, and physical activity and women's health. Dr. Freedson's research interests include the assessment of physical activity; physical activity, fitness, and health in different populations; pediatric exercise physiology; and fitness test development. She has published widely in the scientific literature including several book chapters related to various aspects of exercise physiology. She has been a principal investigator (PI) on grants received from the Centers for Disease Control and Prevention, NIH, foundations, and corporate sponsors. She is a past-president of the Research Consortium of the American Alliance for Health, Physical Education, Recreation and Dance (AAHPERD), and the New England chapter of the American College of Sports Medicine. In 1996, she was the recipient of the Presidential Citation Award from the AAHPERD. In 2001, Dr. Freedson was one of the President's Lecturers at the National American College of Sports Medicine Conference in Baltimore. In 2003, Dr. Freedson delivered the Cureton Fitness Lecture at the American College of Sports Medicine Conference in San Francisco. In 2004, she was the recipient of the Chancellor's Medal and delivered the Distinguished Faculty Lecture at the University of Massachusetts. She is currently Vice President of the American College of Sports Medicine, and a Fellow of the Research Consortium, the American Academy of Kinesiology and Physical Education, and the American College of Sports Medicine.

Glenn Gaesser, Ph.D., is a Professor of Exercise Physiology and Director of the Kinesiology Program at the University of Virginia in Charlottesville. Professor Gaesser was graduated Phi Beta Kappa from the

University of California, Berkeley, where he also received an M.A. and a Ph.D. with a specialization in exercise physiology. His research interests include metabolic and cardiovascular responses to acute and chronic exercise and the impact of diet and exercise on risk markers associated with the metabolic syndrome. He cochaired the writing group that produced the 1998 American College of Sports Medicine (ACSM) position on "The recommended quantity and quality of exercise for developing and maintaining cardiorespiratory and muscular fitness, and flexibility in healthy adults." He is a Fellow of the American College of Sports Medicine, and in the 1990s, he served on ACSM's board of trustees, as chair of its Pronouncements Committee, and as an associate editor of *Medicine and Science in Sports and Exercise*. Dr. Gaesser is also an editorial advisory board member of, and contributing writer to, *Health at Every Size*.

William E. Garrett, Jr., M.D., Ph.D., is Professor of Surgery in Orthopedics at Duke University Medical Center in Durham, North Carolina. Dr. Garrett has a longstanding interest in orthopaedic sports medicine clinical practice and research. He has been especially interested in conditions affecting exercise and performance of the knee, including anterior cruciate ligament (ACL), meniscus, cartilage, and patellar injuries. His clinical activities focus on arthroscopic and reconstructive surgery on the knee and shoulder. He is currently conducting basic and clinical studies on ACL injuries in athletes, particularly to understand the difference between ACL injuries in men and women. He is also working on new instrumentation for ACL reconstructive surgery to create a more anatomic reconstruction with more normal biomechanics. His goal for the Michael W. Krzyzewski Human Performance Laboratory, otherwise known as the K-Lab, is to conduct research in injury prevention and performance enhancement for elite and recreational athletes. Dr. Garrett is past-president of the American Orthopaedic Society for Sports Medicine, and he has served as Director of the American Board of Orthopaedic Surgery. He is also a member of the American Academy of Orthopaedic Surgeons, the American College of Sports Medicine, and an active member of IOC committees. For the past 16 years, Dr. Garrett has served as the Medical Director of the U.S. Soccer Federation, and Chair of the Physical Fitness, Sports Medicine, and Research Committee. He has also served as Team Physician for the U.S. Men's and Women's National Teams in World Cup competition. Dr. Garrett has published widely in the scientific literature, and has edited 13 books and 50 book chapters. He is the recipient of numerous awards, including the

Kappa Delta Award from the American Academy of Orthopaedic Surgeons, the Citation Award from the American College of Sports Medicine, and the George D. Rovere Award for Education in the American Orthopaedic Society for Sports Medicine. He has received teaching awards at both Duke University and the University of North Carolina.

Andrew Goldberg, M.D., is a Professor of Medicine; Chief of the Division of Gerontology; and Director of the Geriatric Research, Education, and Clinical Center (GRECC) at the Baltimore VA Medical Center and the University of Maryland, Baltimore, NIA-NIH Research Training Grant Center in Exercise Physiology and Aging, and the Claude D. Pepper Older Americans Independence Center. He is also Codirector of the University of Maryland Center for Research on Aging. Dr. Goldberg received his medical degree from the State University of New York. He completed his residency at New York University-Bellevue Medical Center and received his fellowship training in the Division of Endocrinology, Metabolism, and Nutrition at the University of Washington in Seattle. He was Assistant Professor of Preventive Medicine and Medicine at Washington University in St. Louis from 1977–1983, Associate Professor and Director of Research in the Division of Gerontology and Geriatric Medicine at Johns Hopkins School of Medicine from 1983–1990, and then became Professor of Medicine at the University of Maryland School of Medicine in Baltimore in 1990, where he established the Division of Gerontology and the Department of Veterans Affairs. Dr. Goldberg leads research programs that investigate the functional declines and medical diseases associated with aging that are influenced by physical deconditioning and factors associated with obesity (lifestyles, genetic, and ethnic factors). Dr. Goldberg's research focuses on the mechanisms by which exercise and weight loss affect and can improve obesity and related metabolic complications. He is currently studying gene-environmental factors that affect fat cell metabolism, particularly lipoprotein lipase (LPL) activity, the rate limiting enzyme for lipid uptake and storage by the fat cell, and the influence of gene polymorphisms (LPL, PPARγ) on metabolic and body fat responses to weight loss and exercise training.

Laurie J. Goodyear, Ph.D., is a Senior Investigator and Head of the Section on Metabolism at the Joslin Diabetes Center, and an Associate Professor of Medicine at Harvard Medical School. She received her Ph.D. in cell biology from the University of Vermont. Her postdoctoral training included fellowships at the University of Vermont, Harvard

Medical School, and in the Section on Metabolism at the Joslin Diabetes Center. Dr. Goodyear is an active member of the American Diabetes Association (ADA), American Physiological Society, and the American College of Sports Medicine. She has served as a member of the NIH Study Sections on Respiratory and Applied Physiology Study and Skeletal Muscle Biology Study. Dr. Goodyear's awards and honors include the Mary K. Iacocca Fellowship from the Joslin Diabetes Center, a New Investigator Award from the American College of Sports Medicine, and Career Development Awards from the ADA and Juvenile Diabetes Research Foundation.

William L. Haskell Ph.D., is Professor Emeritus of Medicine at the Stanford Prevention Research Center. A physiologist by training, his areas of research interests include homodynamic/metabolic effects of exercise; multifactor, intervention, and coronary atherosclerosis; weight loss, nutrition, and exercise effects on lipoprotein and ambulatory blood pressure; and coronary artery disease. Recent work has included exploration of balance, strength, flexibility, and psychosocial effects of different types of exercise training. Dr. Haskell received his B.S. in biological sciences from the University of California at Santa Barbara, his M.S. in exercise science, his Ph.D. in human physiology from the University of Illinois, Champaign-Urbana, and a certification in cardiovascular disease epidemiology from the University of New York at Buffalo. His professional awards include an honorary doctorate of medicine from Linköping University in Sweden; and lifetime achievement awards from the American Association for Cardiovascular and Pulmonary Rehabilitation, the American College of Sports Medicine, and the Council on Aging and Adult Development of the American Association for Physical Activity and Recreation.

Bradley Hatfield, Ph.D., is a Professor in the Department of Kinesiology at the University of Maryland, College Park with adjunct appointments in the Center for Neural and Cognitive Sciences as well as the Center on Aging. He received his Ph.D. in 1982 from the Pennsylvania State University where he was supported by the Research Council of Canada as a doctoral fellow. His research focuses on exercise and the aging brain and the psychological aspects of expert motor performance. This work is characterized by a cognitive neuroscience approach and typically involves neuroimaging of the brain using electroencephalography, event-related potentials, and magnetoencephalography as the primary technical tools. He has published widely in the scientific literature. He is a member of the editorial board of the *Journal of Sport and Exercise Psychology*. Dr. Hatfield's research efforts have been supported by the U.S. Army Research Institute for the Behavioral and Social Sciences, the American Heart Association, the Erickson Foundation, and the Johns Hopkins University Center for Health and Information Technology. He is currently supported by the Department of Defense's Army Research Office, the Army Research Laboratory (Human Research and Engineering Directorate) in Aberdeen, Maryland, and the NIH. Current NIH-supported research is focused on the role of physical activity and genotype in delay of onset of dementia. Dr. Hatfield recently served as President of the North American Society for the Psychology of Sport and Physical Activity and the mid-Atlantic chapter of the American College of Sports Medicine. He is a Fellow of the American College of Sports Medicine, the American Academy of Kinesiology and Physical Education, and a charter Fellow of the American Association for the Advancement of Applied Sport Psychology.

Gregory W. Heath, D.H.Sc., M.P.H., is the Guerry Professor and Head of the Department of Health and Human Performance at the University of Tennessee at Chattanooga, and Director of Research at the University of Tennessee College of Medicine, Chattanooga. Dr. Heath was formally the Lead Health Scientist with the Division of Nutrition and Physical Activity at the Centers for Disease Control and Prevention (CDC). His training is in physiology, nutrition, and epidemiology. Dr. Heath received his M.P.H. and doctor of health science degrees from Loma Linda University in California. He completed his postdoctoral training in applied physiology at the Washington University School of Medicine in St. Louis. A former Epidemic Intelligence Service Officer, he worked at CDC for over 20 years. Dr. Heath has spent most of his professional career devoted to understanding and promoting physical activity and exercise for the enhancement of health and the prevention and treatment of chronic diseases. He has published widely in the scientific literature. Dr. Heath is a Fellow in the American College of Sports Medicine and in the American Heart Association's Councils on Epidemiology and Prevention and Nutrition, and Physical Activity and Metabolism.

Jennifer Hootman, Ph.D., A.T.C., FACSM, is currently an Epidemiologist with the Arthritis Program at CDC. Her research focuses on the epidemiology of musculoskeletal conditions, particularly activity-related injuries and arthritis and other rheumatic conditions, and the relation to physical activity and exercise, function, and disability. Dr. Hootman is an Associate Editor for the *Journal of Athletic Training* and an incoming Coeditor of the *Journal of Physical Activity and Health.* She received her B.S. degree in sports medicine from Marietta College and an M.S. degree in health, physical education, recreation, and dance with a specialization in athletic training from Illinois State University. She received her doctoral degree in epidemiology and biostatistics from the University of South Carolina, focusing on injury and physical activity epidemiology. Dr. Hootman is a National Athletic Trainers Association certified athletic trainer and has worked as a Division I collegiate athletic trainer and undergraduate instructor in sports medicine for 10 years. She is a Fellow of the American College of Sports Medicine.

Bruce H. Jones, M.D., M.P.H., is a Colonel (Retired, U.S. Army) and is currently with the U.S. Army Center for Health Promotion and Preventive Medicine Injury Prevention Program at the Aberdeen Proving Ground, Maryland. He has served on the staff of the U.S. Army Research Institute of Environmental Medicine in Natick, Massachusetts, where he established its injury epidemiology program and was Chief of the Occupational Medicine Division. He has also served as Director of Epidemiology and Disease Surveillance at the U.S. Army Center for Health Promotion and Preventive Medicine and managed its Injury Prevention Program. He has held various positions within the National Center for Injury Prevention and Control at the Centers for Disease Control and Prevention. His research and practice has focused on documenting the effects of injuries on soldiers and military readiness and examining the value of integrated injury and disease surveillance and control programs for the prevention of injuries. Dr. Jones retired from the U.S. Army as a Colonel in July 1998 but continues to consult with the Army and other military services. He is a Fellow of the American College of Preventive Medicine and the American College of Sports Medicine. He received his M.D. from the Kansas University Medical Center in Kansas City and his M.P.H. from the Harvard School of Public Health. He is board certified in preventive medicine.

Wendy M. Kohrt, Ph.D., is a Professor of Medicine in the Division of Geriatric Medicine at the University of Colorado Health Sciences Center in Denver. She is the Director of the Investigations in Metabolism, Aging, Gender, and Exercise (IMAGE) Research Group in the Division of

Geriatric Medicine, and the Director of the Energy Balance Core Laboratory for the NIH-supported Clinical Nutrition Research Unit. Dr. Kohrt's research interests are in the general area of age-related changes in metabolism, sex steroids, and body composition with an emphasis on understanding changes that occur in women after the menopause. Dr. Kohrt's research is focused on understanding why menopause increases propensity for fat gain, particularly in the abdominal region. Her intervention studies involve exercise, weight loss, and/or hormone therapy and focus on the health consequences of abdominal fat accumulation in women and the mechanisms responsible for this menopause-related phenomenon. Another focus of Dr. Kohrt's research is on bone health in aging and the extent to which lifestyle behaviors (e.g., diet and exercise) can protect against bone loss. Current studies are directed at identifying novel factors, such as the use of nonsteroidal anti-inflammatory drugs, which may compromise the benefits of exercise on bone health.

Caroline Macera, Ph.D., is a Professor of Epidemiology at the School of Public Health at San Diego State University (SDSU). Dr. Macera has over 25 years experience as an epidemiologist and has published extensively in the area of physical activity and health. Prior to joining the faculty at SDSU, she led the surveillance and epidemiology team at the Physical Activity and Health Branch at CDC. She also served as Coleader for the *Healthy People 2010* chapter on physical activity and fitness and led the development of the physical activity items that are now used in the CDC's statewide Behavioral Risk Factor Surveillance System.

Richard F. Macko, M.D., is Professor in the Department of Neurology and Medicine, Division of Gerontology; Associate Director of Research for the Geriatric Research, Education, and Clinical Core; and Director of the VA Rehabilitation Research and Development Center of Excellence in Exercise and Robotics in Baltimore. Dr. Frank also serves as Academic Director at the University of Maryland, School of Medicine Rehabilitation Medicine Division, and is a standing member of the (NIH/NICHD) Center for Medical Rehabilitation Research Grants Panel and VA Rehabilitation Research Grant Panels. His research focuses on developing models of task-oriented exercise to improve motor function, cardiovascular fitness, and metabolic health for individuals aging with the chronic disability of stroke. The interdisciplinary approach to this research model includes investigating mechanisms of exercise-mediated neuromuscular adaptations at the central nervous system and peripheral muscular/metabolic levels. Central nervous system investigations characterize brain plasticity in locomotor control of older hemiparetic stroke patients participating in health-promoting treadmill exercise rehabilitation programs that are now shown in randomized studies to improve ambulatory function even decades after stroke. The muscle and metabolic research examines effects of exercise on body composition and molecular mechanisms underlying inflammatory and metabolic abnormalities in hemiparetic muscle, which regulates insulin and glucose metabolism and may be modifiable to reduce recurrent stroke risk.

Robert M. Malina, Ph.D., FACSM, is a Research Professor at Tarleton State University in Stephenville, Texas. He is a former Professor at Michigan State University where he retired in 2002. Dr. Malina's research interests focus on the biological growth and maturation of children and adolescents with an emphasis on motor development and performance, youth sports and young athletes, and the potential influences of physical activity and training for sports. A related area of interest is the growth, performance, and physical activity of Latin American youth with a primary emphasis on Mexico. Professor Malina has served as Editor-in-Chief of the *American Journal of Human Biology* (1990–2002), Editor of the *Yearbook of Physical Anthropology* (1980–1986), and Section Editor for growth and development for the *Exercise and Sport Sciences Reviews* (1981–1999) and the *Research Quarterly for Exercise and Sport* (1981–1993). Dr. Malina also serves on the editorial boards of 13 journals in the sport sciences and biological anthropology. Dr. Malina earned his doctoral degrees in physical education at the University of Wisconsin, Madison, and in anthropology at the University of Pennsylvania, Philadelphia. He has received several honorary degrees (*doctor honoris causa*) from the Catholic University of Leuven in Belgium; the Academy of Physical Education at Jagiellonian University in Krakow, Poland; and the University School of Physical Education in Wrocław, Poland.

Heather McKay, Ph.D., is Professor in the Faculty of Medicine, Department of Orthopaedics and Family Practice, and Interim Director for the Centre for Hip Health at the University of British Columbia in Vancouver, Canada. She is coauthor of two books, *Physical Activity and Bone Health* and *Strong Bones and Muscles,* published by Human Kinetics Publishers. During her eight years at the University of British Columbia, she has published widely in scientific journals about the role of exercise and other lifestyle factors for child and older adult health. Dr. McKay was a Principle Investigator on the development and evaluation of the recently initiated Action Schools! BC—a multidisciplinary, multisectoral physical activity and healthy eating program in elementary schools. This model is a broad-based provincial initiative, supported by three government ministries, which promotes a shift in elementary school culture toward increased physical activity. Action Schools! BC targets cardiovascular health, bone health, obesity, psychosocial health, and academic performance outcomes. Dr. McKay is a Michael Smith Foundation for Health Research Senior Scholar and a Peter Wall Institute for Advanced Studies Career Scholar.

Linda D. Meyers, Ph.D., is the Director of the Food and Nutrition Board at the Institute of Medicine of the National Academies. Dr. Meyers has also served as the Deputy Director and a Senior Program Officer in Food and Nutrition Board. Prior to joining the Institute of Medicine in 2001, she worked for 15 years in the Office of Disease Prevention and Health Promotion in the U.S. Department of Health and Human Services where she was a Senior Nutrition Advisor, Deputy Director, and Acting Director. Dr. Meyers has received a number of awards for her contributions to public health, including the Secretary's Distinguished Service Award for *Healthy People 2010* and the Surgeon General's Medallion. Dr. Meyers has a B.A. in health and physical education from Goshen College in Indiana, an M.S. in food and nutrition from Colorado State University, and a Ph.D. in nutritional sciences from Cornell University.

James R. Morrow, Jr., Ph.D., is a Regents Professor in the Department of Kinesiology, Health Promotion, and Recreation at the University of North Texas. He completed his Ph.D. in Research and Evaluation Methodology from the University of Colorado. His teaching and research focus on measurement issues related to physical fitness and activity assessment and the relationship between these variables and quality of life. He has authored five books and has published widely in the scientific literature. Dr. Morrow has been a coinvestigator on federally funded research projects estimated at approximately $10 million. He has been elected as a Fellow to the American College of Sports Medicine, the American Academy of Kinesiology and Physical Education, AAHPERD Research Consortium, and the North American Society of Health, Physical Education, Recreation, Sport and Dance Professionals. Dr. Morrow has served as Editor-in-Chief of the *Research Quarterly for Exercise and Sport* (1989–1993), and he currently serves as Coeditor for the *Journal of Physical Activity and Health*. He serves as a member of the Cooper Institute's FITNESSGRAM Advisory Board and the President's Council on Physical Fitness and Sports' Science Board.

Miriam E. Nelson, Ph.D., is Director of the John Hancock Center for Physical Activity and Nutrition and Associate Professor of Nutrition at the Gerald J. and Dorothy R. Friedman School of Nutrition Science and Policy at Tufts University in Boston. She holds a Ph.D. in nutrition from Tufts University. For the past 12 years, Dr. Nelson has been the PI of studies on exercise and nutrition for midlife and older adults. Her research is supported by grants from the NIH and private foundations. Dr. Nelson has written several books, including *Strong Women, Strong Bones,* which received the esteemed Books for a Better Life Award for best wellness book of 2000 from the Multiple Sclerosis Society. In 1994, Dr. Nelson was named a Brookdale National Fellow, a national award given annually to five or six young scholars deemed to be future leaders in the field of aging. She was awarded a Bunting Fellowship at the Mary Ingraham Bunting Institute at Radcliffe College for 1997–1998. In 1998, Dr. Nelson received the Life Time Achievement Award from the Massachusetts Governor's Committee on Physical Fitness and Sports. She is a Fellow of the American College of Sports Medicine.

Anne Newman, M.D., M.P.H., is a Professor of Epidemiology and Medicine in the Graduate School of Public Health at the University of Pittsburgh. Dr. Newman has conducted numerous population studies of disease and disability in older adults. As a geriatrician and epidemiologist, she developed protocols to assess functional outcomes (including disability, gait disorders, cognitive impairment) and important geriatric syndromes (e.g., sleep disorders, weight loss) in Pittsburgh's Cardiovascular Health Study (CHS), a 19-year NIH/National Heart, Lung, and Blood Institute (NHLBI)-funded longitudinal study of the risk factors and natural history of cardiovascular disease in older adults. Dr. Newman is the field center PI of CHS ancillary studies including the Sleep Heart Health Study and the Coronary Artery Calcium Study. Dr Newman is the PI of the CHS All Stars, a National Institute of Aging (NIA)-funded study designed to assess exceptional aging and function in the CHS cohort. She is also the PI of the NIA-funded study of Health, Aging, and

Body Composition (Health ABC) at the Pittsburgh Field Center, a longitudinal study of weight change, sarcopenia, and function in an older cohort, now in its 10th year. She is also the PI of the Lifestyle Interventions and Independence for Elders (LIFE) Study, a pilot study designed to assess the feasibility of a full-scale walking intervention trial in healthy and frail older adults. Additionally, Dr. Newman has just been awarded a grant for one of four study centers in the NIA Multicenter Studies in Exceptional Survival in Families, designed to study long-lived families in the United States and Europe. Dr. Newman is Codirector of the Center for Healthy Aging at the University of Pittsburgh, and is also Codirector of the NIA-funded Training Grant in the Epidemiology of Aging. She is the Pilot Studies Core Leader for the Claude D. Pepper Older Americans Independence Center. She has mentored numerous M.D., M.P.H., and Ph.D. students in the epidemiology of aging.

Patrick J. O'Connor, Ph.D., is Professor and Codirector of the Exercise Psychology Laboratory in the Department of Exercise Science at the University of Georgia in Athens. His previous academic appointments include Assistant Professor, University of Georgia, Health and Human Performance, Exercise Science; and Assistant Professor, Arizona State University. He received his B.S. degree in political science from the University of Oregon, his M.S. in exercise science from Purdue University, and his Ph.D. in exercise psychology from the University of Wisconsin. Dr. O'Connor's research has investigated psychobiological and mental health outcomes of acute and chronic physical activity. Dr. O'Connor's research spans several areas, including exploring the influence of exercise on moods such as anger, anxiety, energy, and depression; understanding exercise-related muscle pain by using the R-III nociceptive reflex as a tool to elucidate delayed-onset muscle pain; examining the relationship between physical activity and the human circadian system, including sleep; and understanding the relationship between physical activity and the physical and mental health of very young female gymnasts. He is a Fellow of the American College of Sports Medicine.

Russell R. Pate, Ph.D., is the Associate Dean for Research and a Professor in the Department of Exercise Science at the Norman J. Arnold School of Public Health at the University of South Carolina in Columbia. He received a B.S. degree in physical education from Springfield College, and his M.S. degree and Ph.D. in exercise physiology from the

University of Oregon. Dr. Pate's research interest and expertise focuses on physical activity measurement, determinants, and physical activity promotion in children and youth. He also directs a national postgraduate course that develops research competencies related to physical activity and public health. Dr. Pate is also involved in the CDC funded Prevention Research Center at the University of South Carolina. His research includes studies on preschoolers' physical activity levels and how schools can influence these levels, as well as multicenter trials on physical activity promotion among middle school and high school-aged girls. Dr. Pate serves as an investigator for the Robert Wood Johnson Foundation's Active for Life Program that encourages physical activity among seniors. He serves on the Kraft Food Global Health and Wellness Advisory Council, and is a past-president of both the American College of Sports Medicine and the National Coalition on Promoting Physical Activity.

James Pivarnik, Ph.D., is a Professor of Kinesiology and Epidemiology in the College of Education, Director of the Center for Physical Activity and Health, and Director of the Human Energy Research Laboratory at Michigan State University in East Lansing. His previous academic appointments were in the Department of Health and Human Performance at the University of Houston; Department of Pediatrics and Department of Obstetrics and Gynecology at the Baylor College of Medicine; and Adjunct Associate Professor in the School of Public Health at the University of Texas Health Sciences Center at Houston. Dr. Pivarnik earned his B.S. degree from Indiana University, M.S. degree from James Madison University, and was awarded his Ph.D. from Indiana University. He completed postgraduate training at St. Louis University School of Medicine. As an exercise physiologist and epidemiologist, Dr. Pivarnik studies the exercise responses of females, particularly during pregnancy, and children, both healthy and those with chronic diseases. His focus is on the role of physical activity in reducing the risk factors for chronic disease development (e.g., cardiovascular disease) and the morbidity and mortality of those affected by these conditions.

Judith G. Regensteiner, Ph.D., is a Professor of Medicine in the Department of Cardiology Heart Center, and Director of the Center for Women's Health Research at University of Colorado Health Sciences Center in Denver. Dr. Regensteiner serves on the editorial boards of *Vascular Medicine* and *Diabetes Care*. She is the PI of studies in type 2 diabetes and peripheral arterial disease. Her current research focuses on exercise and type 2 diabetes—gender and endothelial function (funded by the American Diabetes Association) and an NIH-supported evaluation of the mechanisms that explain why exercise rehabilitation is efficacious in treating patients with claudication due to peripheral arterial disease (the AMNESTI study). Dr. Regensteiner is an investigator for two NIH multicenter studies: the Look Ahead trial that is designed to determine whether reducing obesity improves cardiovascular outcomes in type 2 diabetes, and the CLEVER study, which compares the efficacy of angioplasty versus supervised exercise rehabilitation for treating claudication. Dr. Regensteiner has published widely in the scientific literature.

James H. Rimmer, Ph.D., is a Professor in the Department of Disability and Human Development and Adjunct Professor in Movement Sciences at the University of Illinois at Chicago. He also serves as an Adjunct Professor in the Department of Physical Medicine and Rehabilitation at Northwestern University, which is affiliated with the Rehabilitation Institute of Chicago. For the past 25 years, Dr. Rimmer has developed and directed health promotion programs for people with disabilities. He has published widely in peer-reviewed journals and authored several book chapters on various topics related to physical activity, health promotion, secondary conditions, and disability. He directs two federally funded centers: the National Center on Physical Activity and Disability and the Rehabilitation Engineering Research Center on Recreational Technologies and Exercise Physiology Benefiting People with Disabilities. Dr. Rimmer has published standardized measurement instruments that can be used to evaluate the accessibility of fitness and recreation facilities for people with disabilities, and was recently funded by NIH to develop a health empowerment zone for people with disabilities in and around the University of Illinois at Chicago medical campus. Dr. Rimmer is currently completing a CDC-funded randomized trial; the Physician-Referred Community-Based Approach to Increasing Awareness and Sustainability of Physical Activity for Overweight Adults with Mobility Limitations. He is a *Healthy People 2010* Panel Member and was involved in the development of the Chapter 6 Workplan, Disability, and Secondary Conditions. Dr. Rimmer serves on several national committees, including the Scientific and Medical Advisory Board for Life Fitness Academy, and the Executive Committee of the American Public Health Association's Disability Special Primary Interest Group.

RADM Penelope Slade Royall, P.T., M.S.W., is the Deputy Assistant Secretary for Disease Prevention and Health Promotion, and Director, Office of Disease Prevention and Health Promotion, Office of Public

Health and Science, U.S. Department of Health and Human Services (DHHS). She is a Commissioned Corps Officer in the U.S. Public Health Service. RADM Royall leads prevention priorities for DHHS and is a senior advisor to the Assistant Secretary for Health and to the DHHS Secretary. Prior to this appointment, she was Acting Executive Director, President's Council on Physical Fitness and Sports and Senior Public Health Advisor, Immediate Office of the Assistant Secretary for Health. Before joining the Office of Public Health and Science, she was the Chief of Physical Rehabilitation in the Physical Rehabilitation Department, Federal Medical Center, Butner, North Carolina. RADM Royall earned a degree in physical therapy and her M.S.W. degree in social work from the University of North Carolina at Chapel Hill.

David S. Siscovick, M.D., M.P.H., is Professor of Medicine and Epidemiology, Codirector of the Cardiovascular Health Research Unit, and Director of the NHLBI-funded Cardiovascular Epidemiology Training Program at the University of Washington. Dr. Siscovick completed his undergraduate training at the University of Pennsylvania and attended medical school at the University of Maryland before completing a residency in internal medicine and earning an M.P.H. degree in epidemiology at the University of Washington. He was a Robert Wood Johnson Clinical Scholar, a Teaching and Research Scholar of the American College of Physicians, a NHLBI Preventive Cardiology Academic Awardee, and a Donald R. Reynolds Scholar. He is currently a member of the Board of Scientific Counselors of the NIA. He is a clinical-cardiovascular epidemiologist, whose research has focused on the development and application of knowledge related to the prevention of cardiovascular diseases. In addition to his research on the role of exercise and nutrition in sudden cardiac arrest, he has conducted population-based research in genetic, biochemical, pharmacological, and environmental epidemiology related to atherosclerotic metabolic risk and cardiovascular health. He has also contributed to multiple NHLBI-funded prospective, multicenter cohort studies of risk factors, subclinical, and clinical cardiovascular disease, including the Cardiovascular Health Study (CHS), the Multi-ethnic Study of Atherosclerosis (MESA), the Coronary Artery Risk Development in Young Adult Study (CARDIA), and the Women's Health Initiative (WHI). Dr. Siscovick has published widely in the scientific literature, and he is currently the PI of three R01s funded by the NHLBI.

C
Workshop Participants

Katie Clarke Adamson
Director of Health Partnership and Policy
YMCA of the USA
Washington, DC

Brian Armour, Ph.D.
Health Economist
Division of Human Development and Disability
CDC/National Center on Birth Defects and Developmental Disabilities
Atlanta, GA

David Auxter, Ph.D.
Co-Chair, Disability Prevention Task Force
Consortium for Citizens with Disabilities
Washington, DC

David Berrigan, Ph.D., M.P.H.
Biologist
National Cancer Institute
National Institutes of Health
Bethesda, MD

Jennifer Bishop, M.P.H.
Policy Analyst
Department of Health and Human Services
Washington, DC

Steven N. Blair, P.E.D.
Professor
Department of Exercise Science
Norman J. Arnold School of Public Health
University of South Carolina
Columbia, SC

Mona Bormet, M.P.H., C.H.E.S.
Policy Associate
National Research Center for Women & Families
Washington, DC

Barbara Bowman, Ph.D.
Associate Director for Science
National Center for Chronic Disease Prevention, Health, and Promotion
Centers for Disease Control and Prevention
Atlanta, GA

Peter H. Brubaker, Ph.D.
Professor
Departments of Medicine and Health, Exercise Science
Wake Forest University
Winston-Salem, NC

David Buchner, M.D., M.P.H.
Chief, Physical Activity and Health Branch
Division of Nutrition and Physical Activity
Centers for Disease Control and Prevention
Atlanta, GA

Carl Caspersen, Ph.D., M.P.H.
Associate Director for Science
Division of Diabetes Translation
Centers for Disease Control and Prevention
Atlanta, GA

Holly Lea Cintas, Ph.D.
Physical Therapy Research Coordinator
National Institutes of Health
Bethesda, MD

David Conroy, Ph.D.
Associate Professor
Department of Kinesiology
Pennsylvania State University
University Park, PA

Susan Cooper, M.S.N., R.N.
Director, Project Diabetes
State of Tennessee
Nashville, TN

Kerry S. Courneya, Ph.D.
Professor and Chair, Canada Research in Physical Activity and Cancer
Faculty of Physical Education
University of Alberta
Edmonton, Alberta, Canada

Wilma Peterman Cross, M.A.
Senior Program Analyst
National Institute of Arthritis and Musculoskeletal and Skin Disease
National Institutes of Health
Bethesda, MD

Lisa Culver, P.T., M.B.A.
Associate Director
Department of Practice
American Physical Therapy Association
Alexandria, VA

Jesse DeMello, Ph.D.
Associate Professor
Department of Kinesiology and Health Science
Louisiana State University
Shreveport, LA

Rodney K. Dishman, Ph.D.
Professor of Exercise Science and Director, Exercise Psychology Laboratory
Kinesiology Department
University of Georgia
Athens, GA

Joseph E. Donnelly, Ed.D., FACSM
Professor and Director, Energy Balance Laboratory and the Center for Physical Activity and Weight Management
Schiefelbusch Institute for Lifespan Studies
University of Kansas
Lawrence, KS

Bart Drinkard, M.S., P.T., C.C.S.
Physical Therapist
National Institute of Health
Bethesda, MD

Chhanda Dutta, Ph.D.
Chief, Clinical Gerontology Branch
Geriatrics and Clinical Gerontology Program
National Institute of Aging
National Institute of Health
Bethesda, MD

Roger A. Fielding, Ph.D.
Scientist I and Director of
Nutrition, Exercise Physiology, and Sarcopenia Laboratory
Director, Human Studies Jean Mayer USDA Human Nutrition Research Center on Aging
Tufts University
Boston, MA

Sheila Franklin, M.A.
Director
National Coalition for Promoting Physical Activity
Washington, DC

Patty Freedson, Ph.D.
Chair and Professor
Department of Kinesiology
University of Massachusetts
Amherst, MA

Janet Fulton, Ph.D.
Epidemiologist
Division of Nutrition and Physical Activity
Centers for Disease Control and Prevention
Atlanta, GA

Emily Gadola
Public Affairs Research Associate
Trust for America's Health
Washington, DC

Glenn Gaesser, Ph.D.
Professor and Director
Kinesiology Program
Curry School of Education
University of Virginia
Charlottesville, VA

Ewing Garber, Ph.D.
Associate Professor
Northeastern University
Boston, MA

William E. Garrett, Jr., M.D., Ph.D.
Professor of Surgery in Orthopedics
Department of Surgery
Division of Orthopedic Surgery
Duke University Medical Center
Durham, NC

Andrew Goldberg, M.D.
Director, Geriatric Research, Education and Clinical Center
Baltimore VA Medical Center
Baltimore, MD

Laurie J. Goodyear, Ph.D.
Associate Professor of Medicine
Harvard Medical School
Senior Investigator and Head Section on Metabolism
Joslin Diabetes Center
Boston, MA

Molly Greaney, Ph.D.
Research Associate
Harvard School of Public Health
Boston, MA

Kelly Kennai Grunig
Media Relations and Project Manager
YMCA of the USA
Washington, DC

William L. Haskell, Ph.D.
Professor Emeritus of Medicine
Stanford Prevention Research Center
Stanford University School of Medicine
Stanford, CA

Bradley Hatfield, Ph.D.
Professor, Sports Psychology
Kinesiology Department
University of Maryland
College Park, MD

Gregory W. Heath, D.H.Sc., M.P.H.
Department of Health and Human Performance
University of Tennessee
Chattanooga, TN

Jennifer M. Hootman, Ph.D.
ATC Epidemiologist
Arthritis Section, Division of Adult and Community Health
Centers for Disease Control and Prevention
Atlanta, GA

Edward Howley, Ph.D.
Professor
Department of Health and Exercise Science
University of Tennessee
Knoxville, TN

Van Hubbard, M.D., Ph.D.
Director, NIH Division of Nutrition Research Coordination and Senior Advisor to the Secretary
Department of Health and Human Services
Bethesda, MD

Alice Jaglowski, M.S.H., C.H.E.S.
Physical Activity Coordinator
Obesity Prevention Program
Florida Department of Health
Tallahassee, FL

Agnieszka Jarmula
European Commission
Washington DC

Melissa Johnson, M.S.
Executive Director
President's Council on Physical Fitness and Sports
Department of Health and Human Services
Washington, DC

Bruce H. Jones, M.D., M.P.H.
Manager, Injury Prevention Program
Directorate of Epidemiology and Disease Surveillance
US Army Center for Health Promotion and Preventive Medicine
Aberdeen, MD

Geraldine Kennedo
Administrative Assistant
Food and Nutrition Board
Institute of Medicine
The National Academies
Washington, DC

Woodie Kessel, M.D., M.P.H.
Senior Child Health Science Advisor
Office of Disease Prevention and Health Promotion
Rockville, MD

Sue Knaup
Executive Director
Thunderhead Alliance
Prescott, AZ

Harold W. (Bill) Kohl III, Ph.D.
Lead Epidemiologist/Team Leader
Physical Activity and Health Branch
National Center for Chronic Disease Prevention and Health Promotion
Division of Nutrition and Physical Activity
Centers for Disease Control and Prevention
Atlanta, GA

Wendy M. Kohrt, Ph.D.
Professor of Medicine
Division of Geriatric Medicine
University of Colorado Health Sciences Center
Denver, CO

Vivica Kraak, M.S., R.D.
Senior Program Officer
Food and Nutrition Board
Institute of Medicine
The National Academies
Washington, DC

Susan Krebs-Smith, Ph.D., M.P.H.
Chief, Risk Factor Monitoring and Methods Branch
National Cancer Institute
Bethesda, MD

Molly Kretsch, Ph.D.
National Program Leader
Human Nutrition
USDA/Agriculture Research Service
Beltsville, MD

Henry Lukaski, Ph.D.
Assistant Center Director
Agriculture Research Service
U.S. Department of Agriculture
Grand Forks, ND

Caroline Macera, Ph.D.
Professor of Epidemiology
Physical Activity Research Collaborative
San Diego State University
San Diego, CA

Richard F. Macko, M.D.
GRECC Associate Director for Research
Professor
Department of Neurology and Gerontology
Baltimore VA Medical Center
Baltimore, MD

Wolf Maier, D.V.M, D.A.B.T
Counselor, Food Safety
Health and Consumer Affairs
Washington, DC

Robert Malina, Ph.D., FACSM
Research Professor
Tarleton State University
Bay City, TX

Rose Marie Martinez, Sc.D.
Director, Board on Population Health and Public Health Practice
Institute of Medicine
The National Academies
Washington, DC

Heather McKay, Ph.D.
Professor, Faculty of Medicine
Department of Orthopaedics and Family Practice
Interim Director, Centre for Hip Health, Division of Orthopaedic Engineering, Bone Health Research
University of British Columbia
Vancouver, BC, Canada

Kathryn McMurry, M.S.
Senior Nutrition Advisor
Office of Disease Prevention
and Health Promotion
U.S. Department of Health and
Human Services
Rockville, MD

Holly McPeak, M.S.
Nutrition Advisor
Office of Disease Prevention
and Health Promotion
U.S. Department of Health and
Human Services
Rockville, MD

Linda D. Meyers, Ph.D.
Director, Food and Nutrition
Board
Institute of Medicine
The National Academies
Washington, DC

James R. Morrow, Jr., Ph.D.
Professor, Dept. of Kinesiology
Health Promotion and Recreation
University of North Texas
Denton, TX

Miriam Nelson, Ph.D.
Director, John Hancock Center
for Physical Activity and
Nutrition and Associate
Professor of Nutrition
The Gerald J. and Dorothy R.
Friedman School of Nutrition
Science and Policy
Tufts University
Boston, MA

Anne Newman, M.D., M.P.H.
Professor of Epidemiology and
Medicine
Graduate School of Public
Health
University of Pittsburgh
Pittsburgh, PA

Patrick O'Connor, Ph.D.
Professor and Co-Director
Exercise Psychology
Laboratory
Department of Exercise Science
University of Georgia
Athens, GA

Jennifer O'Shea
Director
Dittus Communications, Inc.
Washington, DC

CDR Bernard Parker, M.D.
Office of Commissioned Corps
Force Management
Office of Public Health and
Science, Office of the
Secretary
U.S. Department of Health and
Human Services
Rockville, MD

Russell R. Pate, Ph.D.
Associate Dean for Research
and Professor
Department of Exercise Science
Norman J. Arnold School of
Public Health
University of South Carolina
Columbia, SC

Jim Pawelczyk, Ph.D.
Associate Professor of
Physiology and Kinesiology
Pennsylvania State University
University Park, PA

Cecilia Penn, M.D.
Preventive Medicine Resident
U.S. Department of Health and Human Services
Rockville, MD

James M. Pivarnik, Ph.D.
Professor of Kinesiology and Epidemiology
Departments of Kinesiology and Epidemiology Center for Physical Activity and Health
Michigan State University
East Lansing, MI

Judith Regensteiner, Ph.D.
Professor of Medicine
Department of Cardiology Heart Center
University of Colorado School of Medicine
Denver, CO

James Rimmer, Ph.D.
Director, Center on Health
Promotion Research for Persons with Disabilities
Director, National Center on Physical Activity and Disability
University of Illinois
Chicago, IL

Jennifer Roland, Ph.D., P.T., M.P.H.
Assistant Professor
Department of Disability and Human Development
Center on Health Promotion Research for Persons with Disabilities
University of Illinois
Chicago, Illinois

RADM Penelope Royall, P.T., M.S.W.
Director, Office of Disease Prevention and Health Promotion, Office of Public Health and Science
U.S. Department of Health and Human Services
Rockville, MD

Asel Ryskulova, M.D., M.P.H.
Epidemiologist
National Center for Health Statistics
Centers for Disease Control and Prevention
Hyattsville, MD

CDR Rita B. Shapiro, Ph.D., M.D.
Commander
United States Coast Guard
Washington, DC

Denise Simons-Morton, M.D., Ph.D.
Chief, Clinical Applications and Prevention Branch
National Heart, Lung, and Blood Institute
National Institutes of Health
Bethesda, MD

David Siscovick, M.D.
Professor of Medicine and Epidemiology
Cardiovascular Health Research Unit
University of Washington
Seattle, WA

Christine Spain, M.A., M.S.
Director, Research, Planning, and Special Projects
President's Council on Physical Fitness and Sports
Washington, DC

Pamela E. Starke-Reed, Ph.D.
Deputy Director
National Institutes of Health
Division of Nutrition Research Coordination
Bethesda, MD

Kimberly Stitzel, M.S., R.D.
Science and Medicine Advisor
American Heart Association
Washington, DC

Carol West Suitor, Sc.D., R.D.
Consultant
Northfield, VT

Meredith Terpeluk
Director of Secretarial Prevention Initiatives
Office of Public Health and Science
U.S. Department of Health and Human Services
Washington, DC

Wilma Tilson
Senior Health Policy Analyst
U.S. Department of Health and Human Services
Washington, DC

Beth Topf
Policy Analyst, Prevention
Association of State and
Territorial Health Officials
Washington, DC

CAPT Richard P. Troiano, Ph.D.
Coordinator, Physical Activity Guidelines for Americans
Office of Disease Prevention and Health Promotion
Office of Public Health and Science
U.S. Department of Health and Human Services
Rockville, MD

Jennifer Tucker, M.P.A.
Public Health Analyst
Centers for Disease Control and Prevention
Atlanta, GA

Monica Hobbs Vinluan, J.D.
Senior Policy Associate
National Recreation and Park Association
Washington, DC

Jane Wargo, M.A.
Program Analyst
President's Council on Physical Fitness and Sports
Washington, DC

Richard Weil
Exercise Physiologist
New York Obesity Research Center
St. Luke's Hospital
New York, NY

James Whitehead
Executive Vice President
American College of Sports Medicine
Indianapolis, IN

Mary Wykle, PhD.
Professor, Aquatics Specialist
Northern Virginia Community College and Aquatic Therapy & Rehabilitation Institute
Annandale, VA

Deborah Young, Ph.D.
Associate Professor
University of Maryland
College Park, MD

Judith C. Young, Ph.D.
Vice President for Programs
American Alliance for Health, Physical Education, Recreation and Dance
Reston, VA

D

Acronyms and Abbreviations

ACOG	American College of Obstetricians and Gynecologists
ACSM	American College of Sports Medicine
AHA	American Heart Association
BDNF	brain-derived neurotropic factor
BMC	bone mineral content
BMD	bone mineral density
BMI	body mass index
BRFSS	Behavioral Risk Factor Surveillance System
CDC	Centers for Disease Control and Prevention
CVD	cardiovascular disease
DEXA	dual-energy X-ray absorptiometry
DHHS	U.S. Department of Health and Human Services
FDA	U.S. Food and Drug Administration
GDM	gestational diabetes mellitus
ICF	International Classification of Functioning, Disability and Health
IOM	Institute of Medicine
LDL	low-density lipoprotein

MET	metabolic equivalent
NASPE	National Association for Sport and Physical Education
NCI	National Cancer Institute
NHANES	National Health and Nutrition Examination Survey
NIH	National Institutes of Health
OA	osteoarthritis
RMR	resting metabolic rate
RNA	ribonucleic acid
STRRIDE	Studies of Targeted Risk Reduction Interventions through Defined Exercise
TNF-alpha	tumor necrosis factor-alpha
USDA	U.S. Department of Agriculture
VO_2	oxygen uptake
VO_2max	maximal oxygen uptake
VO_2peak	peak oxygen uptake
YRBSS	Youth Risk Behavior Surveillance System

E

Glossary

Accelerometry In the measurement of physical activity, the use of accelerometers (devices that detect and quantify body movement). Frequently used as a pedometer to count the number of steps taken throughout the day.

Activities of daily living Activities related to personal care that include bathing or showering, dressing, getting in or out of bed or a chair, using the toilet, and eating.

Aerobic capacity (power) An indicator of endurance capacity or fitness. It is a measure of the body's ability to process oxygen. It involves a combination of lung capacity, the size of the capillaries, the pumping action of the heart, and the transfer of oxygen from red blood cells to target tissues. It is frequently referred to as maximal oxygen uptake or VO_2max.

Balance A skill-related component of physical fitness that relates to the maintenance of equilibrium while stationary or moving.

Body composition A health-related component of physical fitness that relates to the relative amounts of muscle, fat, bone, and other vital parts of the body.

Bone mineral content The amount of mineral at a particular skeletal site, such as the femoral neck, lumbar spine, or total body.

Bone mineral density Determined by dividing the bone mineral content by the area of a scanned region.

Cardiorespiratory endurance A health-related component of physical fitness that relates to the ability of the circulatory and respiratory systems to supply oxygen during sustained physical activity. Also called cardiorespiratory fitness or aerobic capacity.

Children Persons ages 2 to 11 years. In this summary, refers mainly to persons ages 6 to 11 years.

Disability A physical or mental impairment that substantially limits or restricts the condition, manner, or duration under which an average person in the population can perform a major life activity, such as walking, seeing, hearing, speaking, breathing, learning, working, or taking care of oneself.

Duration The length of time spent participating in physical activity (e.g., 30 minutes per occasion).

Endurance activities Repetitive, aerobic use of large muscles (e.g., walking, bicycling, swimming).

Evidence-informed The accumulation of data from a wide variety of research designs and clinical experiences used to reach a solid conclusion.

Exercise Planned, structured, and repetitive bodly movement done to improve or maintain one or more components of physical fitness. In this summary, the term is used interchangeably with *physical activity*.

Flexibility A health-related component of physical fitness that relates to the range of motion available at a joint.

Frequency The number of times spent participating in physical activity over a specified period (e.g., two times per week).

Intensity A characteristic of a physical activity that represents how "hard" it is performed or perceived by a person. Examples of intensity categories of a physical activity are light, moderate, or vigorous.

Kilocalorie (kcal) A unit of measurement for energy, either consumed through food and beverages or expended both through physical activity and basal metabolic processes. 1 kilocalorie = 1 calorie = 4,184 joules = 4.184 kilojoules.

Metabolic equivalent (MET) A unit used to estimate the metabolic cost (oxygen consumption) of physical activity. One MET equals the resting metabolic rate of approximately 3.5 ml $O_2 * kg^{-1} * min^{-1}$.

Moderate intensity A general descriptor of the physical activity intensity that causes some increase in heart rate and breathing rate but at which the person feels comfortable exercising for an extended period of time. A benchmark of moderate-intensity activity for a healthy middle-aged adult would be brisk walking.

Muscle fiber An individual muscle cell.

Overtraining The attempt to do more work than can be physically tolerated.

Period The time span that is covered by a survey or other measurement instrument (e.g., the last week).

Physical activity Bodily movement that is produced by the contraction of skeletal muscle and that increases energy expenditure.

Physical fitness A set of attributes or conditions that allows an individual to carry out daily activities without undue fatigue and with sufficient reserve to enjoy leisure pursuits. Physical fitness is assessed through many components, including muscular strength and endurance, flexibility, cardiovascular endurance, body composition, agility, balance, and speed.

Physical inactivity The state of doing no or very little activity (being sedentary).

Power A skill-related component of physical fitness that relates to the rate at which one can perform work.

Resistance training Training designed primarily to increase muscle strength, power, and endurance.

Sarcopenia Age-related degenerative decreases in skeletal muscle mass.

Strain An injury resulting from overstretching and tearing a muscle. A strain can occur through an accident or through improper use or overuse of a muscle.

Strength The ability of the muscle to exert force.

Strength of evidence A general indication of how confident one can be that there is a causal relationship between an exposure (e.g., physical activity) and a specific health or fitness outcome. The strength of evidence will be determined by the number, type, and quality of the studies that have been conducted addressing the relationship, the consistency of the results among studies, and the effect size (or magnitude of the relationship).

Vigorous intensity A general descriptor of the physical activity intensity that causes large increases in heart rate and breathing rate and that causes fatigue within a short period of time. A benchmark of vigorous-intensity activity for a healthy middle-aged adult would be running at 8–10 mph.

VO_2 The amount of oxygen consumed per minute by an individual while performing an activity.

VO_2max The maximal capacity for oxygen consumption by the body during maximal exertion.

Youth Younger and older adolescents or teens, ages 12 to 19 years. For convenience in this summary, the term *youth* is often used to refer to school-aged children and adolescents.